IGNITE!

The Firefly Theory

A Simplified Path to
Your Child's Happiness,
Health and Development

ALDA SMITH

"Firefly, firefly, what makes your light shine?

Is your energy system as complex as mine?

Firefly, firefly, what makes you glow?

Is there perhaps more that we should know?

Firefly, firefly show me the way!

I too want my light to shine bright today."

– Alda Smith, The Firefly Theory

First Edition 2021

978-1-9196199-1-0 – hardcover
978-1-9196199-2-7 – paperback
978-1-9196199-3-4 – eBook

Published by Kinderfli **www.kinderfli.com**

Illustrated by **Elfy Chiang**

Edited by Bridget Lötz **Bridget@lotzpublishing.co.za**

Cover Design by **Studio Stratos**

Typesetting and design by **maguirecreative.com**

To parents of children with special needs: I see you.

To scientists, clinicians and therapists: Thank you for your dedication to the fields of neuroscience, child development, immunology and metabolics. You give parents hope. You inspire me, and I hope that I can do the same for you with this book.

Please feel free to do as many doctorates as it takes to support and even improve on *The Firefly Theory* or theories like it, but be sure to do so in the context of a community. Our ever-growing population of neurodiverse children need scientists, caregivers, teachers, therapists and parents unified in their support. Visit www.kinderfli.com for more information on *You've Got This!* – Kinderfli's Parent Health Literacy Project.

To my beautiful son, Néo: What an amazing person and blessing you are! May you always find your hope in the Creator's providence – knowing that He so governs things that His children will only reap good from whatever befalls them. You are so loved baby bug.

A word on neurodiversity

I have come to know neurodiversity as something to be held in high regard - not merely tolerated. However, due to the distress atypical neurological functioning like ADHD and autism can cause individuals living in a world geared towards the typical, these are still categorised as disorders. I hope that this will one day change, but our children need to be supported in reaching their full potential regardless.

CONTENTS

DNA

NUTRITION

FOREWORD

The human body relies on a magnitude of interconnected cells, body systems and senses — each with its unique function — to serve the universal cause of vitality. Why would things outside the body work differently? In a way, all good things are co-created.

ALDA SMITH, The Firefly Theory

Neurological, mental and immune conditions in children represent a significant and growing burden of disease. According to the World Health Organisation, 10-20% of all children experience mental health conditions such as behavioural disorders (e.g., ADHD); developmental and learning disorders (e.g., dyspraxia DCD, dyslexia and autism spectrum disorder); and emotional disorders (e.g., anxiety and depression). It is estimated that 20% of the world population suffers from allergies. Each year, approximately 400,000 children and adolescents are diagnosed with cancer, which, despite an 80% cure rate, is still the leading cause of death in children from high-income countries.

But why? Why are the numbers growing? Why do we see so many co-occurring conditions in children? Why, despite so many medical advances, do we still not have any concrete answers? How can we prevent and counter adverse developmental and health events in our children?

I would venture that the following are the most significant driving forces behind the escalation in the number of children whose potential is not optimised:
• Changes in our diets and lifestyles.
• The lack of child development and health literacy to adequately deal with these changes.

- The absence of an accepted 'universal truth' in optimising neurological development and immune priming in children.
- The lack of research focusing on the 'invisible' parts of the human body.
- Shortages in appropriate, collaborative support and solutions.

Access to, or selecting appropriate support can also be difficult and overwhelming for parents. With the lack of help comes a growing need for accessible, integrated and collaborative strategies to support disorders and illnesses and the prevention thereof in children.

In the foreword of the World Health Organisation *2006 Report on Neurological Disorders,* Rita Levi-Montalcini (1986 Nobel Prize in Medicine) called for neurological research to be developed in an interdisciplinary way and not in isolation. With this, she not only highlighted one of the biggest challenges in healthcare, but she also left bread crumbs to the following interconnected, universal truth in development and wellness: Just as knowledge and optimised health are co-created in the context of an integrated community, so it is with our different body systems and the energy that they need to function.

In the foreword of her *2018 Annual Report,* Prof Dame Sally C Davies, the Chief Medical Officer of England at the time, gave additional weight to Rita's earlier call by aptly suggesting that all role players in healthcare should work together to develop an environment that would make 'the healthy choice the easy choice.'

I wrote this book to give parents, teachers, and healthcare providers a head start in:
- understanding children's health within a community context.
- understanding health and development in the context of a universal theory.
- understanding health and development as a dualistic outcome of matter and energy or the physical body and energy.
- asking the right questions.

The Firefly Theory highlights the importance of energy system health fundamentals in the prevention and support of neurological conditions, disabilities and illnesses in children – regardless of their genetic make-up. I hope that this book will be the missing, universal truth that will give parents and parents-to-be the agency they need to start the journey of optimising their children's health and development – both before and after birth.

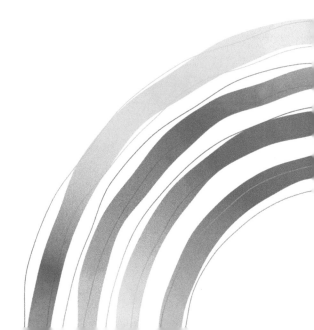

DISCLAIMER

> "I don't believe there would be any science at all without intuition."
> – **Rita Levi-Montalcini, 1986 Nobel Prize in Medicine**

Greetings

Before you start, you must know that I am not a clinician.
I am, however, a dynamic thinker and creative, which means I
understand and often use the discovery potential of my unique way
of thinking. I am also a mother of three children (one with dyspraxia
DCD, apraxia and ADD) and an award-winning, well-published health
and wellness writer and advocate. I have provided emotional support to
over 100 women in labour and birth and have more than 300 hours of
clinical observation experience – including a 20-hour-long paediatric
kidney harvesting and transplant at the Netcare Christiaan Barnard
Memorial Hospital in Cape Town, South Africa. I have developed and
marketed more than one wellness product or device, have completed
training in the Fundamentals of Neuroscience, have a Professional
Certification in Narrative Medicine (which means I have experience in
bridging the gap between the precision of science and messiness that is
life) and have completed basic overview training in photomedicine.

However, I by no means see myself as a scientific expert.

Out of respect for fellow parents, their children and the incredible work
scientists and health professionals do, the plan was at least to have a PhD
under my belt before publishing this book. With the world COVID-19
pandemic of 2020, I, however, realised that there is no better time than

the present and that the future of preventing and treating developmental and healthcare issues in our children, does not lie in another qualification, but instead in a community of parents, teachers, clinicians, scientists, therapists and dynamic thinkers who are willing to serve, collaborate and meet each other as equals. Optimal health is, in my opinion, co-created, and this book is my humble contribution.

The Firefly Theory **is the result of eight years of personal experience and intuitive research, interpretation, simplification, practical application and culling of some of the world's leading experts' knowledge.** It is the discovery and understanding of a universal truth that runs through and connects all the intricacies of health, development and the human body, as well as most of the effective therapies and solutions for childhood disabilities and disease out there.

With this book, I've tried to bridge the gap between the overwhelming complexity of the human body and our ability to make healthy choices based on palatable fundamentals. It is intended as a 'spark', and I hope that it will inspire a culture of hierarchy-free teaching and learning – one where specialists and parents can have meaningful conversations that will ultimately help our ever-growing neuro-diverse population of children reach their full potential. To that end, I have founded the Kinderfli *You've Got This!* Parent Health Literacy Project, which I hope, will, with your help, support parents across the world in the rewarding but challenging journey of raising children and make the healthy choice the easy one. In buying this book, you have already contributed to the initiative in a small way.

Medical Supervision

While this book is based on credible research, lectures, interviews with healthcare professionals and personal experiences, the materials and content are for general information and educational purposes only and are not intended to be a substitute for professional advice, diagnosis or medical treatment. It should always be applied in the context and under the guidance of medical supervision. Nothing in this book should be interpreted as a claim of treatment or cure of any medical condition. Readers should not only rely on the information provided in this book. All specific medical questions should be presented to a qualified healthcare provider.

This book intends to create understanding and knowledge from scientific research in relation to neurological development and immune priming in children. I will attempt to provide you with practical tips and guidelines as to how many neurological and/or immune conditions can be prevented or supported by focusing on cell energy health fundamentals, but none of these guidelines should ever be interpreted as claims of diagnosis, treatment or cure of any medical conditions.

A WORD ON FUZZY
LOGIC AND SCIENCE

> "Science is a way of thinking much more than it is a
> body of knowledge."
> **– Carl Sagan, American Astronomer**

**Intelligence has more to do with how we think and create
meaning from different information and experiences than
about what we know.**

In my experience, there are two kinds of 'thinking': linear or static
thinking, which translates to 1+1= 2 and dynamic or adaptive thinking.
I call the second 'fuzzy logic.' Generally speaking, linear thinking is
associated with science, data and what we can prove, while fuzzy logic is
linked to the humanities, creativity and constructive uncertainty.

Even though it often is the status quo, I think it would be a mistake to
think that one kind of thinking is superior to the other – in fact, they
can't exist in isolation – good science needs both reliable data and fuzzy
logic to create healthy homeostasis. Zora Neale Hurston, an American
anthropologist, hit the nail on the head when she described scientific
research as 'formalised curiosity and the poking and prying with a
purpose.' Adaptive thinking gives us the courage to purposefully brave
uncertainty, while linear thinking grounds our convictions. The one
keeps the other in check. Science is very much the outcome of dualistic
thinking.

Nowhere is this lesson on collaboration, integration and triangulation
better taught than in the developing body and mind of a child with its

dynamic, co-dependent systems. Optimised health is co-created by different body systems and the energy it needs to function, which is why *The Firefly Theory* upholds and requires both linear and adaptive thought.

INTRODUCTION

> "It is only when we are completely lost that we will begin to search for a new way."
> – **Alda Smith, Author of** *The Firefly Theory*

When my son Néo was eight months old, he stopped breathing. I had left him happy, fed and secure in his baby recliner to collect something from the bedroom and was only gone for a couple of seconds when his then three-year-old sister raised the alarm with these four chilling (but life-saving) words: 'Mommy, Néo is blue.'

The animal-like sound that I made as my husband plucked our rigid, eight-month-old son from his recliner came from fear and horror so deep, it still haunts my dreams. I watched my body from afar going through the CPR motions. Check his throat for any obstruction. Nothing. Turn him over on my knee and firmly push him between his tiny shoulder blades. Nothing.

I don't know how I got into the car with him, but I did. I had him on my lap and was doing mouth-to-mouth and compressions as my husband sped to the hospital. Were my chest compressions too hard? Hard enough? He felt like a tiny, limp doll on my lap.

I was screaming and praying so loudly by the time we reached the hospital that a security guard (bless his soul) heard me and came running to open the car door for me. And as the fresh, cold air struck Néo's face, he took his second first breath of life.

But we weren't out of the woods. What followed was a massive seizure. I howled, paralysed in my husband's arms as the ER nurses worked on my baby – his eyes rolled back and his tiny little body twitching in the blue and grey babygrow his granny gave him (I would never be able to look at that babygrow again).

Néo pulled through what was later said to be SIDS-in-the-making. Sudden Infant Death Syndrome is the unexplained death of a seemingly healthy baby under the age of one year. He was hospitalised, prodded and probed. Lumbar puncture. Nothing. Blood tests. Nothing. Another massive seizure. Brain scan. Normal. Heart scan. Normal.

The first round of seizures disappeared as quickly as they came, and we were eventually discharged with no idea as to what had happened or what had caused it.

After that first day and before the age of one, Néo had several more episodes of what was years later diagnosed as symptoms of Sandifer Syndrome (a movement disorder associated with reflux) and three more anoxic seizures. Still, no one could tell us what was causing our little boy's distress. Despite several uneventful EEGs, the doctors put him on an anti-convulsion medicine.

Watching day and night over my child, petrified that he would stop breathing, I spent hours and hours observing him. Convinced that the episodes were a reaction to him experiencing pain, I started doing research and talking to every neurologist and paediatrician who was willing to engage and answer the questions of a desperate, sleep-deprived mother. During a despairing visit to a compassionate homeopath, he told me that Néo was probably suffering from silent reflux. The homeopath had no idea what was causing the episodes and seizures, but he agreed with me that our son was in great pain. I went back to Néo's paediatrician and requested that we look into reflux as a possible contributor to his distress.

One barium swallow later, Néo was taken off the anti-convulsion medication and put onto an anti-acid instead. It was as simple as that – or at least as far as the seizures were concerned. The episodes and seizures stopped – never to return. My research, however, did not. How could something as harmless as reflux cause seizures?

All of my efforts eventually led me to a paediatric neurologist who diagnosed Néo with Reflux-Anoxic Seizures. I had found an answer – to my first question at least.

That was only the beginning. Even though I had a diagnosis, I was compelled to understand what had caused the first year's hell and the dyspraxia DCD Néo would be diagnosed with five years later. I instinctively knew that if I understood his challenges, I could better support this beautiful child and possibly even help others. Little did I know that my journey would eventually lead me to what I view as a universal theory in development and immune priming in children – *The Firefly Theory.*

CHAPTER 1
The Firefly Theory

> "What is easiest to see is often overlooked."
> **– Milton Erickson, American Psychiatrist**

The Firefly Theory **is the universal idea that health and development is the outcome of the dualistic relationship between matter and energy.** It is the quantum-mechanical-chemical perspective that every aspect of a child's vitality and development, even genetic health to some extent, can be traced back to cell metabolism and stimulation and the fundamentals that uphold a healthy energy system within the body.

The theory suggests that optimal development and health are determined by the successful creation, harnessing, and conduction of the energy needed for cell repair, regeneration, growth, connection, and communication within the body – all in an interdependent medley of body systems.

Within *The Firefly Theory* context, a child's energy system health (ESH) is upheld by three key, co-dependent pillars, which we will explore in more detail throughout this book:
- DNA
- Nutrients
- Stimulation

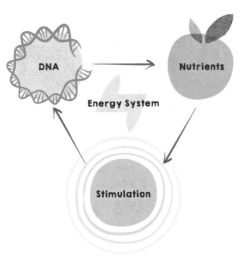

ESH-Triangle

The Firefly Theory works from the calculated position that one can optimise energy system health, and subsequently overall health, within the nervous and other body systems, by understanding how each of the ESH-Triangle pillars plays a role in the creation, conduction, or harnessing and expression of energy. This forms the foundation of providing preventive or therapeutic support to the developing nervous and immune systems in children.

To support the energy system it upholds, there is constant tension and triangulation between the three pillars – the one affecting the other – so that it is hard to definitively say where health and development begin and where it ends. In Chapter 11 – *Pillar Three: Stimulation*, I will venture an educated guess, but what is most important to understand is that like shell, yolk and egg white, all three pillars in the ESH-Triangle are part of the same egg.

Think of a growing child as a plant seedling. If a seedling is not thriving, there could be several reasons – all of which play a role in its energy system health. Perhaps the seed the seedling sprouted from had certain health predispositions (genetics). The seedling might not be getting enough water, oxygen and minerals (nutrients). A lack of sunlight or toxins in the soil (stimulation) can affect how the seedling's genes are expressed, or nutrients are metabolised, which could affect its ability to make and distribute energy needed for optimal growth.

If you follow the domino trail of most disorders or diseases, it will eventually lead you back to one or a combination of pillar dysfunction within the ESH-Triangle. One could go so far as to say that with a pending disease or dysfunction, there is a disturbance in the energy system, but it is not yet visible in the physical body (the preventative nature of *The Firefly Theory* lies within this logic). Illnesses and disorders are really the symptoms of energy system dysfunction and its accumulative, physical effects on the other body systems.

Understanding the ESH-Triangle and its role in overall development and health will provide you with the first outlines of the road map you need to make better choices in support of your child reaching his or her full potential.

You've got this!

The Firefly Theory boils disorder and illness down to the universal idea that if one or more of the ESH-Triangle pillars are negatively affected by lifestyle, diet and/or environmental factors, our children's health and development can suffer.

What does this mean for my child?

The same factors that contribute to disease and disorder serve as the gateway to prevention and support. Understanding the fundamentals of *The Firefly Theory* will help us to:
• ask the right questions.
• make the right lifestyle choices (before, during and after pregnancy).
• make the right nutritional choices (and here we are not only talking about food).
• request the proper tests.
• help us develop integrated strategies with our healthcare providers so that we may optimise the health and development of our children.

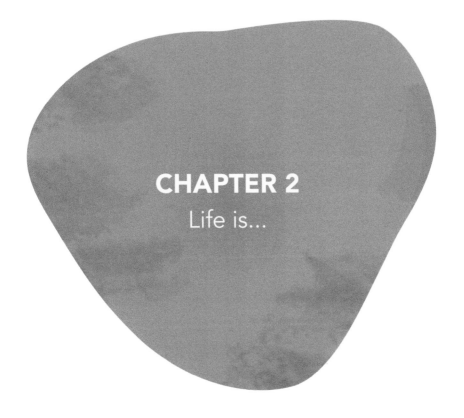

CHAPTER 2

Life is...

"A rainbow is a holographic projection of light through water. Life is a holographic projection of light through our Nervous System."
– **Dr George Gonzalez**, *Holographic Healing*

Physical Body Systems

Modern science describes body systems as physical (chemical or mechanical), interrelated, interactive and interdependent parts that work together to create (and I would add conduct) life. Each body system has a unique function. Like a well-planned machine, the body needs all the systems to work optimally and together to develop and stay healthy.

The twelve physical body systems are:
• The Skeletal System
• The Muscular System
• The Nervous System (brain and nerves)
• The Sensory System (eyes, ears, nose, tongue and skin)
• The Immune System (defence)
• The Cardiovascular System (heart and blood)
• The Respiratory System (breathing)
• The Digestive System (processing food)
• The Endocrine System (hormones)
• The Lymphatic System (drainage)
• Urinary System (kidneys and bladder)
• The Reproductive System

I have already mentioned that these systems are co-dependent, and some of them overlap (the immune and the digestive system, for example). Still, we will discuss these (the nervous and immune systems in particular) in more detail in later chapters.

The Energy System

Probably one of the most overlooked body systems in modern science is the energy system. Ironically, the manifestation of the energy system is the collective purpose of all the other physical body systems. By the same token, the energy system enables, maintains and influences (through metabolism and stimulation) all other biological body systems and, therefore, life.

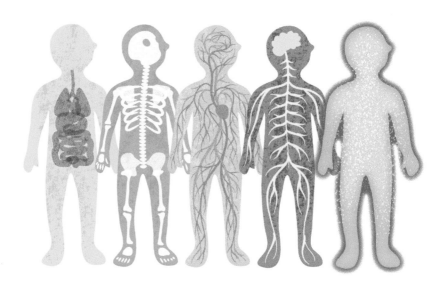

If the physical body systems form the cogs of a machine, then the energy system provides the power and parts required to build, repair and operate that machine. It not only creates the energy we need to live, but it also facilitates the building and maintenance of the very structures through which that energy is conducted or expressed.

Any living body simultaneously contains physical body systems and an energy system.

In his paper, *The Scientific Hypothesis of an 'Energy System' in the Human Body*, Tianjun Liu describes the relationship as being similar to a physical shape that will always have an inextricably linked shadow. "Brain cells are visible, but consciousness is not," he continues.

In theory, the energy system is intangible. It cannot be directly observed or measured. It can only be expressed through the other physical body systems, which might explain its Cinderella status in a world where science is, by its very nature, synonymous with linear thinking.

Studying the energy system can, to use C.S. Lewis's words, be compared to 'taking your eyeballs out to see your eyes.' But even though it is difficult to 'scientifically demonstrate' the energy system, scientists actually use its existence in medicine. Magnetic Resonance Imaging (MRI) reads the vibration or energy of the cells and tissues to create imaging. The electroencephalogram (EEG) is a scientific test that uses energy to measure brain metabolism and activity.

In science, energy is defined as the ability to produce change, do work, or move, while the harnessing of energy for regulation and reproduction (in other words, to do work) classically describes life. Understanding the correlation between these two definitions opens up a whole new area of life science – one that is focused on the 'invisible' parts of the body like quantum neurology. 'Invisible Life Science' may bring forth the elusive universal theory we need to support our children in reaching their full health and developmental potential.

In his book, Holographic Healing, Dr George Gonzalez talks about life being a 'Holographic LightBody' expressed through our physical bodies – the nervous system in particular. I would build on this by saying that life is energy created, harnessed and expressed by our interconnected physical and energy body systems to reproduce, regulate and do work. To that end, we can say that all diseases and dysfunction have their beginning in the body's energy system.

Some of you might experience a 'Eureka!' moment at this point, but don't despair if you still feel confused. Much like the 3D image hidden in a stereogram, *The Firefly Theory* may only become visible after looking at the grainy pattern for a long time - adjusting the way your eyes perceive information.

You've got this!

Having employed many therapies to support Néo in his delayed development, I found photobiomodulation (light therapy), electrotherapy and sound therapy to be of immense value when used in combination with other treatments and specific lifestyle and dietary changes. In my quest to understand what the correlation between these therapies and changes was and why they only seemed to have a positive outcome when applied in combination, I discovered the energy system, the ESH-Triangle that upholds it (DNA, nutrients and stimulation), as well as the three key ingredients that ultimately determine health or dysfunction: nutrition, lifestyle and environmental factors.

What does this mean for my child?

Optimum health and development are determined by the health of our energy system and the cascading impact it has on our other body systems. For our children to reach their full potential, we need to understand the energy system, the pillars that uphold it and the areas in which we can preventatively or therapeutically contribute to this system.

Even though Néo's seizures were, therapeutically speaking, the focal point after his first episode that fateful day, I would later discover that they were but a symptom, albeit a terrifying one, of a perfect storm that had been brewing for some time, perhaps even from before he was born. An invisible energy storm upheld by DNA, nutrition and stimulation – before and after his birth.

CHAPTER 3

A Quantum-Mechanical-
Chemical Perspective

"If atoms, the smallest unit of matter, consist of energy swirling around a nucleus, it would not be a leap to conclude that function and dysfunction; health and illness are a matter of energy – or should I perhaps say, an energy of matter!"
– **Alda Smith, Author of *The Firefly Theory***

The Energy System at Work

It goes by different names - a 'gut feeling,' 'vibe', 'aura', or 'sixth sense'. In a linear context, all of those ideas refer to the vibration of a living organism – an energy system at work. Organisms like plants and animals use energy vibration to communicate. It is speculated that a seizure alert dog can recognise a scent that its partner gives off before a seizure. Scent is a chemical energy that vibrates at a particular frequency. Humans can sense vibrations as well – some more so than others – but overall, our awareness of it seems to have faded with the development of language and other communication skills. So, where does this energy vibration come from?

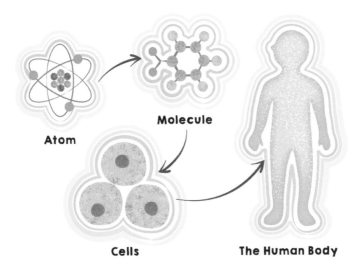

Molecule

Atom

Cells   **The Human Body**

The smallest unit of physical matter, called an atom, consists of an energy force field created by electrons and neutrons, swirling around a nucleus, causing the atom to vibrate or move in a certain way at a particular energy wave frequency. Atoms make up molecules – each vibrating at its unique frequency. Physical matter consists of molecules. An example of this is the large molecule compounds called proteins that form the physical building blocks of our human cells. Like the atoms they are made of, each kind of protein and cell in our body has a specific shape and 'vibrational fingerprint.' For example, different kinds of neurons fire at different frequencies, creating a vibrational language unique to each type. These vibrations create interactive energy waves.

Constructive and Destructive Interference

When the energy waves of two different entities meet, like the ripples of two stones being dropped into water, the waves will meet and interfere with each other. Such interference can either be in sync (in-phase or constructive interference) or out of sync (out of phase or destructive interference). Whether constructive or destructive interference is positive or negative depends on the desired outcome – so don't let the terms confuse you when trying to apply what you've learned to your child's health and development. Alpha energy waves with frequencies between 7 and 13 hertz are, for example, associated with mindful or resting brain frequencies, whereas Beta to Gamma frequencies of between 13 and 40 hertz are associated with the frequencies of an engaged brain ready for problem-solving.

Constructive interference creates more powerful energy waves. When an opera singer hits a high note that vibrates at the same frequency as a certain kind of crystal glass, the in-phase sound energy waves can become so powerful that the glass can break. It has been speculated that hit songs all have very specific constructive frequencies that resonate with our own and that good music is, in fact, a mathematical or scientific wonder.

Waves that are out of phase deplete energy. Noise-cancelling headphones use destructive interference to cancel out loud sounds. It picks up on the sound wave coming in and then sends its own, shifted sound wave to cancel out the noise.

It is the reality of energy wave interference, both constructive and destructive, that lies at the heart of scientific research into electromagnetic pollution and how modern technologies, like mobile phones, affect our health. It also plays a role in many therapies for health and development, including light therapy, electromagnetic therapy, sound therapy, aromatherapy, and occupational therapy. More about this in Chapter 11 - *Pillar Three: Stimulation.*

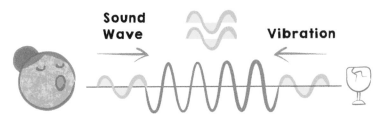

Sound Wave   **Vibration**

Constructive Interference

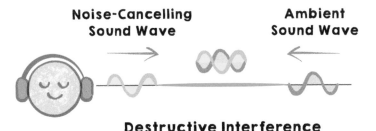

Noise-Cancelling Sound Wave   **Ambient Sound Wave**

Destructive Interference

You've got this!

The human body exists of matter (molecules and cells) that vibrates at specific frequencies – such frequencies determine the shape and function potential of the molecules and cells. This phenomenon is very eloquently explained by Dr Bruce Lipton in his book, *The Biology of Belief.*

The Firefly Theory defines energy wave interference – constructive or destructive – as stimulation. The differently shaped protein molecules in the human body are like the cogs in a machine. With their unique 'vibrational fingerprints' and shape, they have the potential to move and create a particular behaviour or function. Still, they need the right kind of interfering stimulation to harness and use their energy.

What does this mean for my child?

A child's health and development start and end with energy. This energy is created, harnessed and expressed by a physical (mechanical and chemical) body of systems.

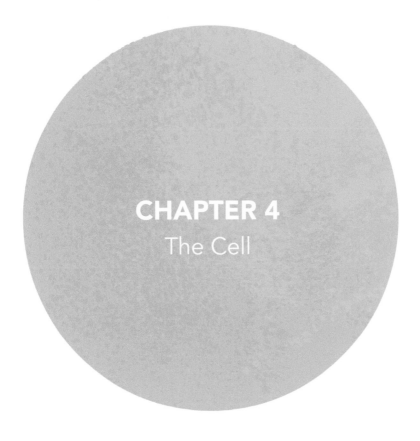

CHAPTER 4
The Cell

"With the discovery of the cell, biologists found their atom."
– **Francois Jacob, Nobel Prize-winning Biologist**

To understand and apply the universal fundamentals outlined in *The Firefly Theory*, **you must understand what constitutes the minimal living unit through which energy is created and expressed - the human cell.**

All living organisms, from single-celled bacterium to multicellular organisms, like humans, are made up of cells. Cells are the smallest living units constituting life. In fact, every human is actually a community of cells working together. Understanding how cells work can help you understand your developing child better – allowing you to prevent certain health events and provide better support when challenges occur.

Cells come in many sizes and specialised shapes (depending on their protein molecules) and can live from one day (white blood cells fighting infection) to a lifetime (some nerve cells in the brain). Cells are the living building blocks of the 'physical' human body. Different types of human cells carry

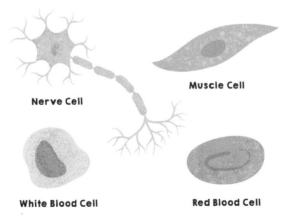

Muscle Cell

Nerve Cell

White Blood Cell   **Red Blood Cell**

out various functions related to homeostasis (body balance regulation) – depending on the tissue and body system they make up. Red blood cells look like doughnuts and carry nutrients like oxygen. The nerve cell is long with 'tentacles' and carries electrical signals. Muscle cells can contract and relax for motor function.

Inside the Cell

Each human cell is made up of chemical molecules, which can be roughly broken down as follow:

- 64% water
- 16% protein
- 16% lipids (fats)
- 4% minerals and carbohydrates

This ratio already hints at the importance of certain food nutrients and why protein and lipids are often called the 'building blocks of the body', but more on that later.

The cell membrane, consisting of proteins and lipids, encircles the cell and controls what enters and exits. Just like a body with systems and organs, the

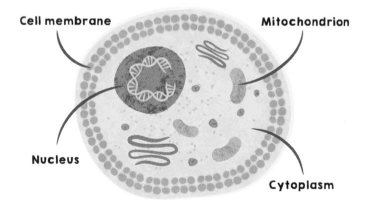

The Human Cell

cell has organelles that float in the cell's cytoplasm – a jelly-like fluid made up of water and nutrients. In fact, the cell within its membrane has all the body systems' functions (e.g., metabolism, respiration and waste removal). Of the different organelles, the nucleus (home to our DNA) and the mitochondrion (the cell's powerhouse) are probably most relevant for this book. We will explore them in more detail over the following two chapters.

The Cell's Job

The cell is the physical embodiment of the invisible energy system. Like a modern-day city, it holds the potential to create, harness and direct energy – vibrating with life.

In addition to its typical cellular functions, cells also have differentiated, specialised functions during which energy is used to do the specific job a cell is intended for in relation to the body. Red blood cells, for example, carry oxygen from the lungs to the rest of the body. A neuron uses energy in the form of electrical pulses or signals to send messages to and from other cells and body systems. Stem cells, also called master cells, can, like the Joker in a card game, use energy to change into more than 200 different types of cells and specialise in those cells' functions, which is why they are so important in terms of staying healthy and repairing damaged tissue or organs.

The Cascading Effect of Cell Damage or Loss

Cell damage or inappropriate loss does not only compromise the body's ability to produce energy (whether in that particular area or another), but the physical impairment or absence can also affect the optimum harnessing and conduction or expression of energy in other cells. Therefore, a broken arm not only means broken physical tissue, which has an impact on the immediate area, but it can also affect other areas. Similar to a blown bulb in a string of festive lights, a damaged or obstructed cell can put out the light in otherwise healthy cells as well.

This cascading effect of cell damage or loss is even more relevant when it comes to cells that have a function directly linked to energy production and conduction. If someone loses a lot of blood during surgery, the body's ability to bring oxygen to other cells might be compromised. Similarly a tethered spinal cord that is stuck or fixed to the spinal canal can cause many metabolic and stimulatory dysfunctions.

You've got this!

Cells create energy to create more energy, create and repair the cells through which the energy is conducted, do the work the cell is intended for, and uphold the energy system.

The physical cell and the energy it creates and needs are entirely co-dependent. Like an object that can't lose its shadow, one cannot exist without the other. So, where should our efforts to prevent adverse health events start? Where should you look if your child's physical body, which is made up of cells, shows signs of dysfunction or illness? The answer is undoubtedly cell energy health.

What does this mean for my child?

When a child presents with an illness or dysfunction, the symptoms can be so overwhelming that we don't know where to start. To support a child effectively, we need to break both health and disease down to its smallest origin – the cell.

The cascading effect of inappropriate cell damage or loss on energy system health might also, in part, explain why children with neurological or mental challenges, like autism spectrum disorder (ASD), for example, so often have additional conditions like allergies co-occurring with the primary condition. *It was only when I realised this truth that I was able to, for example, link an inexplicable and chronic rash on Néo's little chin to his other challenges and effectively treat it.*

CHAPTER 5
The Mighty Mitochondria

"Mitochondria are to a cell, what the brain is to the nervous system – the **power station** of a city."
– Alda Smith, Author of *The Firefly Theory*

At the heart of the body's energy system lies a set of physical and chemical reactions, which together with stimulation are responsible for the 'living state' of cells. We call this breaking down of molecules or blending of compounds for the production, harnessing and expression of energy, **metabolism**.

Metabolism

The main purposes of metabolism are:
- Converting nutrients into energy for all cellular functions. This includes typical cellular functions like more energy production, cell repair and cell death, and specialised cell functions like oxygen transportation.
- Converting nutrients (primarily proteins and lipids) into the cell and DNA building blocks, which can be used in cell structure, growth, repair and multiplication.
- Converting nutrients into or use them as cell energy stimuli (including signalling molecules like hormones and neurotransmitters or catalysts like enzymes), immune helpers (like antibodies), and cell cleaners (like antioxidants and water).

Mitochondria are sausage-shaped organelles inside the human cell that act as their metabolic power stations. Depending on the energy requirement of the tissue or organ, the cell can have from one up to

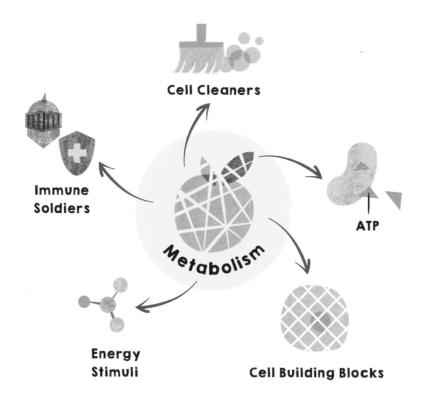

Cell Cleaners

Immune Soldiers

ATP

Metabolism

Energy Stimuli

Cell Building Blocks

1,000 mitochondria. The heart and muscle cells, for example, need a lot of energy and therefore would have more mitochondria in their cells. Almost like a 'cell within a cell,' each mitochondrion has its own membrane and **DNA**.

Most Important Job: Producing Cell Energy

The mitochondria in our cells provide us with the majority of Adenosine Triphosphate (ATP) our energy systems need. ATP is an essential extracellular signalling molecule that acts as the currency of biological energy in the body and is necessary for all metabolic processes and cellular functions. The mitochondria create it by synthesising **glucose**

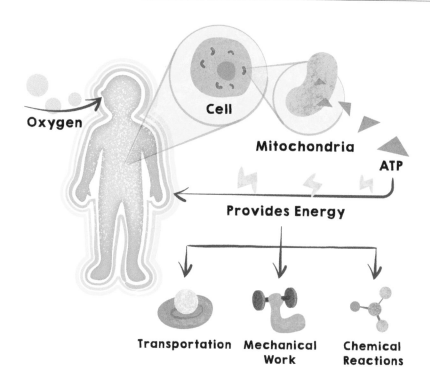

Creating ATP through Cellular Respiration

molecules (which come from the food we eat) and **oxygen** (which comes from breathing) in a process called cellular respiration. The energy released from ATP is used for substance transportation, mechanical work, and chemical reactions. Substance transportation is important for removing toxins, the concentration of ions and the generation of charges to send signals. ATP is also converted into kinetic energy, which the body needs for the heart to pump, blood to circulate and muscles to contract. The chemical energy derived from ATP is used to synthesise molecules.

There is a photoreceptor or a membrane protein called Cytochrome c oxidase on the inner membrane of each of the mitochondria in our cells. It has many functions, one of which is to 'receive' **light photons** (from the sun, for example) and **electrons**, which in turn **stimulate** the last step in the cell respiration process. This is an example of why stimulation from outside the body (e.g., light) plays an important role in energy system health. More on that in Chapter 11 – *Pillar Three: Stimulation.*

Multi-tasking

Mitochondria are also involved in other metabolic and cell processes.

• Just like the body creates waste after digesting food, mitochondria create a by-product called Reactive Oxygen Species (ROS) – also known as 'free radicals' – when synthesising ATP. ROS is commonly known for cell damage and oxidation.

• Generally speaking, the cell nucleus, home to our DNA, is considered the 'brain' of the cell. In a way, this role is, however, shared with the mitochondria – with the nucleus providing the 'cortex' of the cell and the mitochondria providing the 'energy brain.' Messages, called mitochondrial signalling, are sent by the mitochondria to the cell nucleus - instructing which genes in the cell DNA should be expressed and which ones should be switched off. More on this in Chapter 6 – *Pillar One: DNA.*

• The mitochondria oversee cell death when the time is right. Recent studies suggest that they even maintain lysosome structure and function (lysosomes are the repair and waste centres of the cell). This is of particular relevance in cancer, where altered or compromised mitochondria can play a role in the rapid and stubborn spreading of cancerous cells.

You've got this!

In this chapter, we only scratched the scientific surface of the mitochondria, but the goal of *The Firefly Theory* is to make the healthy choice, also the easy one for parents. To this purpose, the concepts most relevant to the theory have been highlighted:

- metabolism; power stations
- DNA
- glucose; oxygen
- stimulate (light photons; electrons; free radicals)

It might still seem very grainy, but the first outlines of the ESH-Triangle and how it might contribute to our children reaching their full potential should start appearing now. I would encourage you to revisit the previous chapters until you feel comfortable with the concepts explained, as the following chapters will be dedicated to an in-depth look at each of the ESH-Triangle pillars: DNA, nutrition, and stimulation.

What does this mean for my child?

When Néo first showed some motor development and co-ordination delays, his neurologist ordered some blood tests for metabolic disorders, which he subsequently tested negative for. At the time, I didn't understand the connection between metabolism and my child's delays. It was only years later, when I discovered the importance of mitochondria and the metabolic processes they drive, that I understood the reason for the tests.

To better prevent and support adverse health events or developmental challenges in our children, we need to reverse-engineer their health to the ESH-Triangle within the human cell and the pillars that uphold it: DNA, nutrition and stimulation.

A NOTE OF ENCOURAGEMENT FROM THE AUTHOR

DNA

Before you start the next chapter, I thought it important to close the science books for a moment and talk to you from the heart – parent to parent. For many obvious reasons, genetics can be a thorny and emotionally charged topic – for some, more so than others. Within them lies the gift of diversity, the potential for incredible joy, but also the possibility of gut-wrenching pain.

We want our children to be happy – not to suffer. This means that things that seem out of our control, like DNA, scare us. As a parent of 14 years, I have, however, discovered that if you can't learn to parent from a place of humility – understanding that you can't control everything – you can become a hot mess of stress, worry and anguish. Don't even get me started on the (mostly self-inflicted) guilt trips! Too much destructive stress does not do anyone or anything any favours – least of all DNA. Learning how to do what you can, and embrace what you can't, is a journey in loving your children for who they are while helping them grow into their full potential. As parents, we are the gardeners – we can support our sprouting seedlings, but we can't control the weather or turn a tomato plant into kale. Besides – do we really want to?

The Firefly Theory intends to help you with the 'what you can do' and the 'helping them reach their full potential' parts. Still, I would be amiss if I didn't acknowledge that there are aspects of our children's health and development beyond our control as parents. Coming to terms with that reality looks different for different people. I'm not going to be as presumptuous as to try and give advice. All I will say is this: I see you, my fellow gardener.

In writing this chapter and trying to scientifically explain concepts that will empower you to support your child, words like 'mutation,' 'damage,' 'disease', and 'faulty' were inevitable. Don't let these words be hurtful or scary – they are linear – not dynamic. As a mother of three vastly different children – one with learning and developmental challenges – I can tell you that, except for a handful of devastating genetic conditions (and even perhaps then sometimes with enough grace), it is often the 'mutated' gene that leaves you belly-laughing with your child. Sometimes it is the 'faulty' gene that renders you speechless as it offers you a new window with a magnificent view and sharp perspective. It can be the 'damaged' gene or extra chromosome that, in fact, makes you whole and gives you courage and compassion you never knew you had.

With that in mind, let's get gardening!

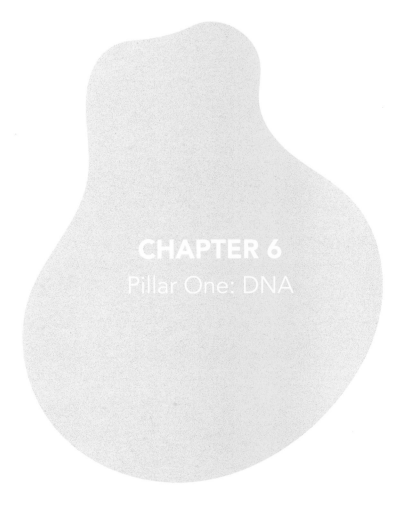

CHAPTER 6
Pillar One: DNA

DNA

> "Genetics is like a family recipe book collection, passed down from generation to generation – each generation updating the collection by adding or culling books and scribbling their own footnotes and adaptations to the remaining recipes."
> **– Alda Smith, Author of *The Firefly Theory***

We know that most of our traits are inherited from our ancestors through DNA. But what is the role of DNA in health and development, and is this molecule our children's only destiny?

Chromosomes, DNA and Genes

Inside every nucleus of a human cell, you will, in most instances, find 46 chromosomes that come in 23 pairs. One exception is in the sperm and ova, which carry only one copy of each chromosome. These will merge to make 23 pairs of combined chromosomes during fertilisation.

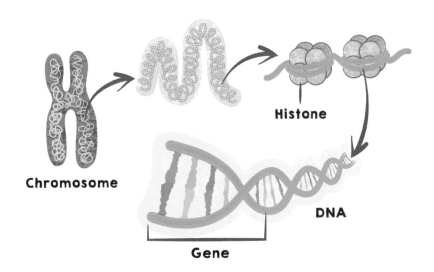

Histone

Chromosome

DNA

Gene

Of the 23 pairs of chromosomes, only one pair will determine gender – females have two X-chromosomes in this pair, and males have one X- and one Y-chromosome. The remaining 22 pairs will determine the physical body and other characteristics, but not gender.

Chromosomes consist of deoxyribonucleic acid molecule chains (DNA) that are tightly wound around protein molecules (histones) – similar to fishing line wound around a reel. This is so that all the DNA chains can fit into the cell's nucleus. If the DNA chains in a cell are laid out in a line, they could be between 1 and 2 m long! The protein in DNA not only acts as the reels. They have another important function, which we will examine when we discuss gene regulation and modulation.

Our DNA has segments that provide coded cell instructions, called genes. We inherit our genes from our parents, who inherited their genes from their parents.

DNA Function

Our DNA provides the recipes or blueprint for our physical cells and their creation, harnessing and expression of energy.

In other words, the two main functions of DNA are:
• to provide a genetic blueprint to ensure that the next generation of cells are 'built' precisely the same.
• to provide instructions or 'recipes' for the creation of different proteins from amino acids that will be used as cell building blocks, cell energy stimuli, immune helpers, or cell cleaners – depending on the proteins' sequence, shape and energy frequency.

The DNA of a human cell has the 'recipes' to more than 80,000 different proteins needed in structural or energy-related processes within the cell.

But how does this relate to our children's development and health? Think of it as knitting something warm for your little one to wear. The kind of clothing you will knit and how it will look and feel will greatly depend on the pattern you use. Now, of course, other things will play a role too – the kind and quality of the yarn you use, the size of the knitting needles, and so on, but it all starts with the pattern. A child's structural or energy-related patterns (DNA) will always lead the metabolic processes and stimulation, ultimately determining development and health. Nutrition and stimulation are also vital (more than we think, as we will learn in the next chapter), but DNA is the starting point.

The Mitochondria DNA

As we learned earlier, the 46 chromosomes in the nucleus do not form the only blueprint or recipe book collection in the cell. Each mitochondrion in the cell also has its own DNA chain with instruction genes or 'recipes' that mainly relate to energy production. Although there can be duplicates, not all of the mitochondria in a cell have the same genome or 'recipe books.'

Interestingly the mitochondrial DNA (and, in fact, all our mitochondria organelles), unlike the nucleus DNA, always comes from a baby's mother. I've often wondered if this fact can partially explain the prevalence of chronic fatigue syndrome or 'yuppie flu' (hypothetically linked to

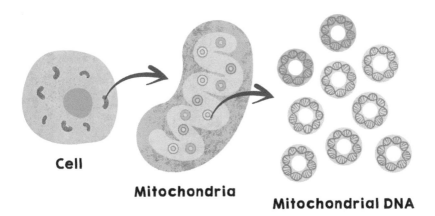

Cell

Mitochondria

Mitochondrial DNA

mitochondria dysfunction) in women. However, it is clear that when we think about the genome our children inherit, we can't only consider the DNA that they inherit from both their mother and their father. We also need to consider the mitochondrial DNA (mtDNA) inherited from their mothers only.

Mitochondrial DNA is more fragile than the DNA in the nucleus, making it highly susceptible to mutations and damage. In fact, the accumulation of mtDNA damage or mutations throughout your life is thought to play an important role in the process of ageing. This could perhaps, in part, explain why, with older mothers, the risk of DNA-related disorders in babies can be higher – perhaps more so than with older fathers.

Dysfunction of the mitochondria can be caused by its own defective mtDNA genes or those expressed by faulty genes in the nucleus DNA (the expression of which are sometimes 'ordered' by the mitochondria through mitochondrial signalling). Several inherited and acquired diseases are linked to dysfunctional mitochondria or mtDNA, e.g., Alzheimer's disease, Parkinson's disease, cancers and diabetes.

Because there is more than one mitochondrion in a cell, you can have both healthy and faulty mitochondria. The impact of the faulty mitochondria and whether it will be collectively expressed as a primary mitochondrial disease (i.e., directly impacting a cell's ability to produce ATP) will depend on how many of them there are. Given the critical role of the mitochondria, it should come as no surprise that primary mitochondrial diseases, characterised by a disruption of the ability to produce ATP, can be devastating.

The Impact of DNA on a Child's Developmental and Health Destiny

It is clear that without the correct structural and energy-related recipes from both the nucleus DNA and the mitochondrial DNA, our bodies would not be able to make and harness energy productively, and without productive energy expression, there is no life.

By the same token, faulty DNA recipes can, if expressed or used, compromise energy creation and conduction, which can lead to cascading illness, dysfunction, and developmental delays in our children.

Nucleus and Mitochondrial DNA Faults

To understand how DNA can be modulated to help our children reach their full health and development potential, it is important to understand the following about DNA faults:

- Both nucleus and mitochondrial DNA faults come in the form of damage or mutation. Damage is an abnormal DNA molecule structure, and mutation is a change in the standard molecule sequence. DNA faults can, to an extent, be repaired, but there are ones that are permanent.

- The reason damage or mutation in a gene can be a problem is that it changes the protein recipe (i.e., the amino acid combinations and sequencing). When a protein recipe changes, it changes the shape and the way the protein vibrates. It also changes the way the protein will move or act (i.e., its function) when stimulated via constructive or destructive interference (see Chapter 3 – *A Quantum-Mechanical-Chemical Perspective*).

- Nucleus DNA faults, whether by damage or mutation, can be inherited – from either or both parents. This means that both the genetic and lifestyle health of the mother and the father comes into play when a baby is conceived. It is already a well-known fact that women who smoke during pregnancy put their babies' health at risk. A study by

Professor Diana Anderson from the University of Bradford's Division of Medical Sciences, however, also found a strong correlation between DNA damage in the sperm of fathers who smoke and DNA changes in their newborn babies.

• Inherited mitochondrial DNA faults come from a child's mother only.

• DNA faults can also be acquired, e.g., through smoking, excessive alcohol, ROS or free radicals, ageing, physical or emotional trauma, UV-radiation, viral or bacterial infections and errors occurring during cell replication.

• An acquired DNA fault in the mother or father can be inherited by their child, as well. This suggests that children can literally 'inherit' trauma experienced by their mothers (or fathers if the acquired fault lies within the nucleus DNA).

Some DNA faults can be fixed, but whether healthy or compromised, fixable or unfixable, your child's DNA is not his or her only health and development destiny. DNA manifestation can be modulated with the help of the other two ESH-Triangle pillars - nutrition and stimulation.

CHAPTER 7
DNA Regulation and Modulation

> "Genes get turned on, turned off or modified by our environment,
> what we eat, who we surround ourselves with and how we
> lead our lives."
> – **Lynne McTaggart, Author of** *The Intention Experiment*

Nature vs Nurture

The "nature or nurture" debate is one of the oldest discussions in psychology. It refers to whether we behave and who we become is determined by our genome or our experiences and environments. We can also apply this to our mental and physical health and abilities.

In his book, *Disconnected Kids*, Dr Robert Melillo writes about two studies on the cause of autism in children. The first study from 1997 involved eleven identical and ten fraternal twins, in which one sibling of each twin had autism. The second Stanford University School of Medicine study was conducted in 2011 on 192 pairs of identical and fraternal twins, of which at least one in each pair had autism.

The first study found that the probability of the second sibling developing autism was significantly higher in identical twins than in fraternal twins, concluding that autism and other neurobehavioral disorders are caused by genetics. However, the second study provided convincing evidence that environmental factors are actually more at play than genetics in determining whether a child will develop autism.

Prior studies had estimated an autism risk contribution ratio of 90/10 (90 being genetics and 10 being environmental factors). However, the Stanford University School study shows that genes only account for 38% of autism risk, compared to 62% for environmental factors.

So which is it – nature or nurture? The answer is nearly almost both. Yes, a child will not get autism if the 'recipes' or genes for its 'creation' are not present. Still, it is also possible that a child who carries the recipes for the structural or energy-creating metabolic processes needed to 'express' autism never ends up having autism.

If Health is Co-Created, then so is Adversity

You might have noticed that I wrote in the plural form when referring to the genes that cause autism. That is because many a-typical manifestations are not single-gene manifestations. There is, for example, no one gene mutation that results in autism. Researchers have instead found that there are hundreds of different gene mutations that, if expressed, can manifest as autism. That is also why, like many other developmental challenges, autism is hard to diagnose and support and why it is classified as a spectrum condition – meaning that there is variation in the type and prominence of the symptoms or traits children with this condition display.

Despite the important role DNA plays in our children's energy system, and therefore overall health and development, it is clear that a gene rarely acts on its own – other genes, nutrition, and stimulants almost always play a role. It is in this accumulative reality, expressed by *The Firefly Theory's* ESH-Triangle, that parents' power to prevent and support dysfunction and adversity lies – and not only because DNA is not the only pillar in the triangle, but also because the two other pillars – nutrients and stimulation – can be applied to prevent inherited DNA faults from being expressed.

Remember the knitted garment? It turns out that the kind of wool and needles not only contribute to the overall knitwear, but it can play a role in determining which pattern will ultimately be knitted from and how the pattern will be read.

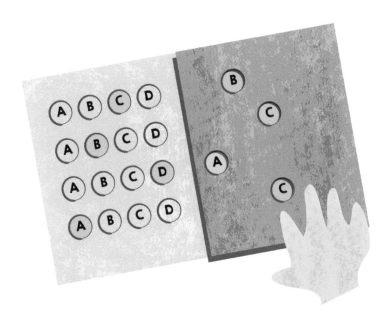

DNA

Epigenetics: Our Golden Ticket (or Stencil) to DNA Modulation

Not so long ago, scientists believed that our genes were set in stone – that they were the ball-and-chain that every person inherited – something that could not be influenced or changed. This meant that our DNA provided a forecast of our health destiny and that we had little control over the diseases and dysfunction that might befall our children or us.

A new area of scientific research called epigenetics is, however, disproving this theory. Epigenetics refers to DNA modifications that do not affect the DNA sequence, but rather which genes in the DNA are 'on' or 'of' – expressed or not expressed.

Remember the exam scoring stencils teachers used to mark multiple question answers before everything became digital? The stencils had small window sequences that would only show the correct answers when placed over the answer sheet. Epigenetics work in much the same way, with nutrition and stimulation determining the 'stencil sequence' known as the cell's 'epigenome' (meaning 'upon genome').

Physical proof that this invisible 'gene stencil' exists, lies in our different body parts. Have you ever wondered how there could be such diversity in the shape and function of our ears, eyes, and organs if most of our cells have the same DNA or cell building block recipes? Different cells express different gene recipes, i.e., some genes are 'switched on' and some genes are 'switched off'. Epigenetics also plays a role in stem cell activation and differentiation, which is important in repairing and healing the body.

Our genome library contains thousands of different protein recipes in each cell. This is why our DNA molecules are wound around the protein reels – so that all these recipes they have can fit into each chromosome. We need all of the recipes for energy system health, but not simultaneously. A cell's function is determined by which genes are 'on' and the shape, vibrations, and ultimate function of the proteins being created from the 'expressed' genes. During development and later on in life, a child's DNA accumulates chemical marks created by how nutrients and other chemical and physical signals 'interfere' with the proteins in DNA. This process is called methylation. Like the scoring stencil, these marks determine which genes are open or closed off – switched on or off. These epigenomes determine gene expression and can change whether a gene releases its recipe instructions and how it is interpreted.

Not to be confused with DNA mutation or damage, epigenome governs the expression or silencing of DNA – both healthy and faulty. This explains why a child may have the genes associated with autism but never develop autism. Recent research shows ways to reverse the closing or opening of unfavourable windows in the epigenome. Still, prevention through genetic regulation and modulation is more obtainable.

Dr Bruce Lipton, the author of *The Biology of Belief*, summarises epigenetics as follows: "Epigenetics doesn't change the genetic code; it changes how that's read. Perfectly normal genes can result in cancer. Vice-versa, in the right environment, mutant genes won't be expressed. Genes are equivalent to blueprints; epigenetics is the contractor."

DNA Regulation and Modulation

DNA faults, whether damaged or mutated, can be inherited – from either or both parents. This means that both the genetic and lifestyle health of the mother and the father comes into play when a baby is conceived.

The epigenome (the DNA stencil) of a human is fluid and is constantly changed by factors relating to nutrition and stimulation. These changes can last from hours to a lifetime. This fluid quality of epigenetics allows us to say that our children's DNA is not their only health and developmental destiny.

When a cell divides (like when a child grows), its epigenetics are passed on to the next group of cells. This does, however, not happen within reproductive cells – almost giving the cell a 'clean epigenome slate' during reproduction. The parents' 'stencils' guide the first epigenetic changes of the fertilised egg. As the embryo develops, it will take over this role. The 'environment' of an embryo to a large extend determines the epigenetics of a baby at birth. That is why a pregnant woman's environment and behaviour during pregnancy play such an important role.

Examples of negative stimulation and nutritional influences include:	Positive stimulation and nutritional influences include:
• environmental toxins • pathogens like certain viruses and bacteria • food with high sugar contents • stressful events like emotional trauma or surgery	• phytonutrients • positive experiences • healthy lifestyle choices • targeted therapies

Connecting with *The Firefly Theory*

In this chapter, we have learned about DNA and its role, but what are the health implications for our children?

Here's how you can connect with DNA's role in the ESH-Triangle:

1. Knowledge is power. Understanding the role of DNA in accumulative energy system health (or dysfunction) will guide you in which aspects of DNA you can regulate and modulate and how to do it. It anchors our understanding of health and development and helps us not waste valuable energy by being confused and fearful.

2. Understanding the role of genetics in our children's development and health can guide us in our choices of healthcare support and the strategies to prevent and counter adverse developmental and health events.

3. Understanding the role of DNA in development and health can guide our questions and help us to understand diagnoses. It can also help us to better analyse the risk and benefits of certain treatments.

4. Understanding DNA can support us in family planning and guide our lifestyle choices both before and during pregnancy.

A SECOND NOTE OF ENCOURAGEMENT FROM THE AUTHOR

> "Guilt is a food group all on its own, and it's the only one I advise everyone to remove from their diet."
> — **Jordanna Levin,** *The Inspired Table*

If, like me, you've earned some stripes in the battle of nutrition, I permit you to omit a heavy sigh at the prospect of this next chapter – let it out of your system. Most of us know of the ancient Greek physician Hippocrates's sentiment that food should be our medicine. He was, of course, right, but what was a simple enough health strategy 2,500 years ago has, due to environmental and lifestyle changes, become complicated and almost impossible to navigate.

Not only has the quality of our food changed, but today we are so overwhelmed by the sheer volume of information, advice, and clutter in child nutrition that, despite our best efforts, we often find ourselves confused and misinformed - reaching for the nearest bag of crisps in utter exhaustion.

The food industry is not making it any easier on parents either – and here I'm not just talking about the confectionery and snack market that left the bag of crisps in my line of sight at checkout. Time is money – which is why fast-food and unhealthy staples are cheap and plentiful. Many parents can't afford to feed their children, let alone provide healthy, balanced meals.

The nutritional food markets are not always innocent either. Not only is it not consistently inclusive in terms of the many price, convenience, allergy, taste, sensory and environmental considerations parents of the 20th century are saddled with, but the market is saturated with confusing and empty promises. Add a picky (or as I like to say 'tricky') eater, time constraints, baffling food labels and a lack of nutrition literacy to the mix, and you have yourself a powder-keg of frustration and food fatigue. As a parent of more than one tricky eater, I have been there, done that and have the cupboards overflowing with half-used supplements and food fads to prove it.

I'm not undermining the importance of nutrition in energy system health – it's vital – but the last thing any modern-day parent needs is another non-organic, fast food shaming exercise (guilt and stress are bad for our health, remember). Instead, this next chapter is focused on helping you separate the wheat from the chaff by explaining the role of nutrition in the ESH-Triangle. Once you understand the 'why' of nutrition, it will, together with a pinch of gratitude, a dash of good humour and some 20th-century food sense, help you make food – not war. Leaving all judgement at the kitchen door is a prerequisite – food choice shaming wreaks havoc within the ESH-Triangle.

Lao Tzu, a Chinese philosopher, once said, "Give a man a fish, and you feed him for a day. Teach a man to fish, and you feed him for a lifetime." The goal of the next chapter is to teach you 'how to fish' (or 'how to grow a veg garden' if you are vegan) so that if your child can benefit from a metabolic evaluation and therapeutic diet, you will know what to ask nutritional specialists and have a guiding light in interpreting the advice given. It can also just support you in developing your own customised nutritional strategy – one that helps you make the best of the resources available to you and works for your family.

CHAPTER 8
The Chapter before Nutrition

"No nutrient in the body works alone."
— **Alda Smith, Author of** *The Firefly Theory*

In Chapter 3 – *A Quantum-Mechanical-Chemical Perspective,* **we saw that the human body consists of molecules that vibrate at a particular frequency and that the frequency of a protein molecule, for example, determines the shape and function potential of that molecule.** This means that nutrients in our body have the potential to do certain things for us, but they need to be stimulated into final shape, movement or action and function.

That is why we need to look briefly at stimulation before diving into nutrients – stimulation being when two or more energy fields interfere with one another. For that purpose, we will be focusing on the stimulation that happens within the gut, by means of gut flora, because that is the point of entry for most nutrients. Our friend Hippocrates was not wrong when he said, "All disease begins in the gut."

Our immune system, which is – as we will later learn – also one of the most important endo-stimulation systems in our body, is made up of different cells, soluble and organs, such as the skin and digestive tract. If you consider that the gut makes up 75-85% of the immune system and that many, if not most inflammatory diseases originate from here, it makes sense for parents to make gut health a priority when it comes to their children.

We all have gut bacteria or flora that help with the breakdown and absorption of all nutrients needed while making certain toxins, poisons, dangerous bacteria and viruses stay away. If unbalanced, the bacteria in the digestive system cannot do their job properly. This can lead to malnutrition and a compromised immune system.

Babies are born without the required gut bacteria. Soon after birth, a baby's digestive system is colonised with its mother's blend of digestive flora. A baby can 'inherit' an unbalanced or disturbed flora balance from its mother. This fact in itself makes a strong case for the promotion of a healthy flora balance in pregnant women. But what is an 'unbalanced gut flora'?

Understanding the Unbalanced Gut

An unbalanced gut in its simplest form can mean that there are not enough good bacteria in the digestive system to activate white blood cells and other important functions.

But, according to Dr Patrick Nemechek, author of *The Nemechek Protocol for Autism and Developmental Disorders*, it can also mean that microbes that should live in the more alkaline colon have over-grown the bacteria living in the more acidic small intestine. This is called bacterial overgrowth or SIBO. SIBO can influence cell behaviour in many ways. It can cause cells to produce acid, toxins or stimulate reactions to certain foods like milk or tomato (food allergies or sensitivities). This happens because fragments of the bacteria cells (called LPS) can leak into the bloodstream (called 'leaky gut'). LPS compromises the function of cells, like the microglia that repairs and prunes neurons in the brain. Leaky gut can also stimulate the release of excessive cytokines (signals or messengers that causes inflammation) into the body or trigger excessive production of propionic acid – an ethane-comprising fatty acid that, according to Dr Nemechek, is partially to blame for some serious neurological disorders. Parasites and unwanted microbes in the gut can also disturb cell behaviour.

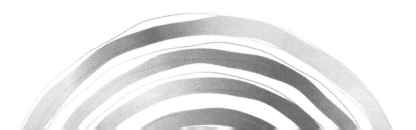

Symptoms of an Unbalanced Gut

Gut health seems to be affected by a highly complex process, which happens on a microscopic level, so how can parents and carers know if a child's microbial is disturbed? It's not always obvious.

Symptoms of unbalanced gut flora in children can include:
• reflux
• heartburn
• food allergies
• eczema
• constipation
• diarrhoea
• neurological symptoms like developmental delays
• lower febrile seizure threshold in children

But there may be problems without any symptoms, and pregnant women or new mums who suspect they might have flora imbalances or suffer from any inflammatory conditions or diseases should be especially mindful of their babies' flora balance and additional outside stressors.

From a more scientific perspective, some laboratories can analyse stool samples to determine overall gut health.

Rectifying a Disturbed Gut Flora

Before you run for the nearest immune boosters and supplements on the shelf, it is important to note that priming your child's immunity can be as important (if not more critical) as boosting it. A disturbed digestive system cannot absorb nutrients properly, and simply adding supplements can be like putting a plaster on an open wound.

We must look at feeding our digestive and immune systems well before looking at nutrients for the rest of the body.

Feeding the Digestive and Immune Systems

- Make sure your child gets the right amount of good fatty acids (Omega 3).
- Avoid oils with excessive amounts of Omega 6 (they can be pro-inflammatory).
- Dr Nemechek recommends a good prebiotic like inulin to balance an unbalanced gut. He explains that a good prebiotic will feed the bacteria in the small intestines and make it too acidic for the colon bacteria to overgrow and cause SIBO.
- Avoid excessive amounts of carbohydrates (excessive carbohydrates paralyse white blood cells, as we will see later on).
- Make sure that you include fermented foods in a child's diet. It will add beneficial probiotics and enzymes to the digestive system.
- Be aware of positive and negative endo- and exo-stimuli or signals (called stressors). We will learn more about these in Chapter 11 – *Pillar Three: Stimulation.*

When I think back on Néo's inexplicable reflux-anoxic seizures, the fact that SIBO can cause lower seizure thresholds and is promoted by strong antacids sometimes makes me wonder about my own gut flora at the time of his birth. Feeding his digestive system well has contributed to many improvements, and today, I am grateful to say that he is seizure and allergy-free.

Prevention is Better than Cure

A new mum can make sure that her baby's gut flora is optimised by looking after her own digestive system during pregnancy and breastfeeding. Mums who choose to feed their babies with formula milk are encouraged to be mindful of milk formula labels and ingredients.

Balanced Nutrition

The next chapter is written from a preventative and maintenance point of view only. Therapeutic diets are highly specialised and should be implemented under the guidance of a clinician to address specific dysfunction and disease in children. However, if you have a child who needs additional support, you will still find the information helpful, as it will guide you to ask the right questions and evaluate solutions with your care provider. It will also help you see how nutrition is but one pillar within the ESH-Triangle – never acting alone in dysfunction or illness.

NUTRITION

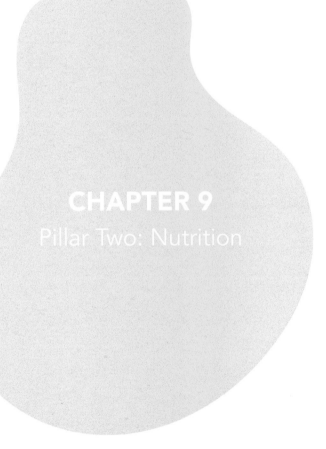

CHAPTER 9
Pillar Two: Nutrition

> "The food you eat can be either the safest and most powerful form of
> medicine or the slowest form of poison."
> **– Ann Wigmore, Holistic Health Practitioner and
> Raw Food Advocate**

What qualifies as nutrition?

Not everything we eat or drink can be classified as nutritious.
The Oxford Dictionary defines food or nutrition as 'any substance that
provides nourishment essential for maintaining life and growth.' The
World Health Organisation defines malnutrition as 'deficiencies, excesses
or imbalances in a person's intake of energy and nutrients.'

The Firefly Theory defines nutrition, one of the key pillars of the
ESH-Triangle, as any substance that provides the raw metabolic
fuel or potential needed to produce energy, DNA and cell building
blocks, cell energy stimuli, immune helpers, or cell cleaners.

NUTRITION

Achieve Balance with Nutritional Objectives

When preparing a meal or a drink for a child (or yourself), it is helpful to
know the nutritional objectives for that meal and its order of importance
beyond addressing hunger pangs. To that purpose, the following five
questions are very helpful:
• Do I need it to provide fuel (glucose) for energy (ATP)?
• Do I need it to provide cell building blocks for both the brain and
  body?
• Do I need it to support the production or activation of cell
  energy stimuli (including signalling molecules like hormones or

neurotransmitters and catalysts like enzymes)?
- Do I need it to prevent or repair cell or DNA damage by supporting and regulating the production of antibodies and inflammation signals for fighting germs and irritants?
- Do I need it to prevent or repair cell or DNA damage by helping the body get rid of free radicals, toxins and irritants?

Of course, all of the objectives are important, but you won't necessarily be addressing all of them with each meal. Understanding your child's dietary goals can make balanced nutrition a lot easier and less stressful to navigate.

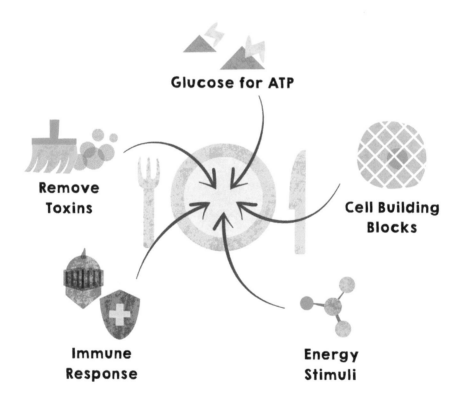

Glucose for ATP

Remove Toxins

Cell Building Blocks

Immune Response

Energy Stimuli

Nutritional Objectives

For some parents with tricky eaters, it might also be helpful to at first try and balance these objectives in the context of a week and not a day. However, keep in mind that nutrients that are almost single-handedly responsible for cell metabolism, like water and enough glucose, are of daily importance. I specifically say 'enough' glucose as too much of any nutrient can have as many negative health implications as too little.

We will deal with other qualifying questions for healthy, balanced and effective nutrition over the next sections.

Every Child is Different

Next, you should look at ratios, intake frequencies and portion sizes. If you grew up between the 70s and 90s, you would remember the 'food pyramid,' which was an effort to provide a guiding light in balanced nutrition and ratios. Today we know that it was deeply flawed in its over promotion of complex carbohydrates and attack on protein and even fat.

A more trustworthy starting point in understanding deficiencies, excesses, or imbalances is, in my opinion, the nutrient ratio in the human cell from Chapter 4 - *The Cell:*
- 64% water
- 16% protein
- 16% lipids (fats)
- 4% minerals and carbohydrates

It is, however, imperative to remember that developing children have different energy needs than adults or someone trying to lose weight. The younger a child, the bigger or more regular the carbohydrate ratios will be, for example. Age, gender, and specific metabolic requirements of children need to be considered.

Once you understand the functions and ratios of food, you can fine-tune your choices by keeping the following in mind:

Nutrients work better in Teams

Given the whole premise of this book, I'm sure the idea of nutrients needing each other is not novel. Nutrient synergy happens if one nutrient helps a person to absorb another. An example of this is the need for vitamin D to absorb calcium. Nutrient synergy also refers to the fact that certain nutrients work better in combination to achieve a nutritional goal. One example is the need for oxygen in producing ATP from glucose, which is why exercise is so important.

Another example of such a 'dynamic duo' is vitamin B12 and L-methylfolate (many know it as folic acid, but we will get to that). These two nutrients work together to support cell division and replication, and yet many pregnant women are only advised to consider their folate intake during pregnancy.

Some nutrients might also reduce the absorption of others. For example, high doses of zinc can reduce the amount of copper absorbed, which is why copper should be taken with zinc to avoid depletion.

Sorting out which nutrients go with which is something stressed-out parents should not have to concern themselves with. But who or what will step up to the plate and ease our burden? The foods on our shelves fortified with nutrients? Nutritional supplements with isolated nutrients? Like with most things, mother nature knows best. Whole food does most of the heavy lifting and calculations for us by providing perfectly balanced nutrient complexes.

Whole Foods vs Processed or Refined Foods

Whole foods are not processed at all (like vegetables and fruit) or processed minimally (like cooked eggs or legumes). From the moment food is altered from its original raw state, it starts losing nutritional value. For example, nutrients will begin to lose their potency when heated over 49 degrees

Celsius. Most processed or refined foods were exposed to temperatures far exceeding that and contain synthetic or isolated chemicals to put back nutrients and flavours and preserve the food for longer. In *Holographic Healing*, Dr George Gonzalez refers to these kinds of foods as 'phudes.'

When selecting food for a child, it is important to know the difference between 'phude' and food. The easiest way to do this is to ask whether the food will recognise itself as something that occurs naturally on this planet when looking in the mirror. Phudes, like sugar and some nutritional supplements, will have a serious identity crisis!

Also, be on the lookout for the phudes dressed up as foods – better known as genetically modified (GM or GMO) or Frankenstein foods. These are foods that are created in laboratories by crossing species that cannot cross in nature. GM foods promote the transfer of antibiotic-resistant genes, but their consumption can also interfere with the epigenetic process.

In *The Metabolic Approach to Cancer*, by Dr Nasha Winters and Jess Higgins Kelley, GM foods are pinpointed as one of the main culprits in the explosion of breast cancer since its introduction in the 1990s. The book points out that the rate of other diseases, such as immune disorders and celiac disease, also increased with the arrival of GM foods like wheat and other grains with gluten proteins.

According to the Center for Food Safety in the U.S., up to 92% of U.S. corn is currently genetically modified, as are 94% of soybeans and 94% of cotton (cottonseed oil in food products).

Beneficial Processing

Food preparation and processing can have either a positive or negative impact on food and is an essential consideration in nutrition. We've already learned that, more often than not, less is more when it comes to food processing, but that certain foods, like eggs, have to be cooked for safety and other reasons. We also know that from 45 degrees Celsius onwards, the nutritional value of food will start to change. This is why slow cooking or poaching at lower temperatures is often viewed as better cooking options than boiling or frying.

Irradiation is a kind of radiation that dramatically increases the shelf life of both fresh and ambient foods. Its destructive energy interference with food kills the bacteria that spoil foods. Still, it also affects the presence of enzymes that aid in our digestion and nutrient absorption of that very food.
Enzymes are, like gut flora, metabolic stimuli. When can food processing then be beneficial?

The germination of grains and plant seeds, also called sprouting, can make it more gut-friendly, break down antinutrients like phytic acids and gluten, as well as increase nutrient levels. Sprouts are, however, often linked to cases of food poisoning, so if you would like to include them in your child's diet, it is important to ensure that they come from a reputable source, that you store them in a dry and cool location and that you wash them in cider vinegar and water before serving them. If you're still worried, you can also slow cook them. Sprouted grain flours can also be a healthier alternative to regular flour, which means more nutritious bread without concern for food poisoning.

Fermentation is another food process that our children's diets can benefit from. Through fermentation, yeast can partially break down gluten in sourdough bread. The lactose in fermented dairy, like yoghurts, is also broken down. Fermentation adds beneficial probiotics and enzymes to food.

Absorbing Nutrients

One area of nutrition often overlooked is a child's ability to metabolise and absorb the nutrients from their meals. We call this the bioavailability of the nutrients.

Technically nutrients that the digestive system has not absorbed are not 'in' our bloodstream and cells yet. Apart from water and oxygen, your child can only benefit from nutrients when digested and absorbed. There are a couple of ways to improve this process.

It all starts with chewing. The 'finer' food is chewed, the easier it is absorbed. Human saliva also contains enzymes that help with the breaking down of food. Chewing properly can be a challenge for children with oral sensitivities. Mashing or pureeing food for them is one way to help them absorb the nutrients while you gradually introduce them to other food textures and sensations.

In *Disconnected Kids,* Dr Robert Melillo notes that children typically have a limited amount of food they will eat because they have yet to define their sense of smell and taste. He says that children who do not smell or taste very well, judge food by texture. To that purpose playing 'smelling games' can improve your child's eating habits as well. Slow and steady is the key point to remember.

Most of the actual absorption of nutrients does not happen in the stomach but in the small intestine. Here are a couple of ways to improve the bioavailability of nutrients for your child:

- Whole foods are the best starting point for the bioavailability of nutrients because of the nutrient synergy in food complexes.
- We've seen earlier that we need certain 'nutrient pairs' for better absorption (like L-methylate and vitamin B12).
- Healthy fats, like olive oil, can help with the absorption of certain nutrients.
- Phytic acids in grains, seeds, and other plants can inhibit the absorption of nutrients like calcium and magnesium. Sprouting is one way of dealing with this issue. Another is not to consume sources of calcium, like milk, with plants.
- Fermentation can help with the breakdown of lactose and gluten.
- Certain antioxidants, like the carotenoids in tomatoes and carrots, are better absorbed when cooked.

NUTRITION

The Blood-Brain Barrier

Chapter 12 – *The Nervous System* will discuss the nervous system in detail, but for this section, it is important to note that children's brains have very different nutritional needs compared to their bodies. Unlike the cells in the body mostly made up of protein, brain cells consist primarily of lipids. This also means that the brain, which needs a lot of glucose, gets most of its glucose from carbohydrates and not fat.

When you want to measure the nutrient deficiencies in the brain, you can't do so by drawing blood. Unlike other cells, most neurons cannot be replaced, so the brain needs extra protection. To keep toxins and pathogens out, the brain relies on a membrane that lines the brain's blood vessels. This membrane is called the blood-brain barrier (BBB). The membrane has small 'gaps' that
allow molecules, like nutrients, to leave the blood vessel to reach the brain tissue. Because the gaps are smaller in the brain's blood vessels, only molecules of a particular size can fit through. Certain chemicals (like alcohol) and pathogens can, however, still cross the barrier to the brain, which is why taking alcohol during pregnancy can be so destructive to a developing foetus's nervous system.

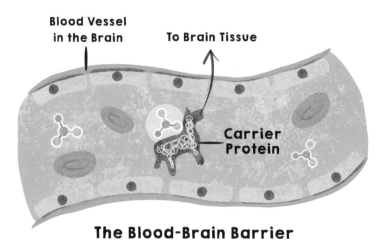

The Blood-Brain Barrier

Let's look at an example of how the blood-brain barrier is relevant to nutrients. Children who do not produce enough of a neurotransmitter called serotonin can struggle with low mood, anxiety, or sleep. Serotonin is metabolised in the brain from an amino acid called tryptophan. There could be many reasons for serotonin deficiencies – one being the recipe (gene) it is made from (serotonin is a protein) and how it is interpreted.

Because of the blood-brain barrier, low serotonin levels in the brain can't be boosted by oral or intravenous supplementation. The tryptophan molecules needed by the brain to produce serotonin from are also too big to cross the blood-brain barrier on their own. They need a 'carrier protein' to get them through – almost like The Trojan Horse entering the city of Troy. To make it even more complicated, 'The Trojan Horse' struggles to enter the city if there are too many other proteins competing with it. This means that a diet that is too high in protein can reduce tryptophan crossing into the brain. Carbohydrates, on the other hand, triggers the production of insulin that helps The 'Trojan Horse' along. This means that a child with a serotonin deficiency can benefit from eating foods that are high in tryptophan and carbohydrates (e.g., pumpkin seeds).

Meat is also a source of tryptophan, but it might not be the best choice if you're looking for a meal to boost the crossing of tryptophan in the brain because it is high in protein.

It is important to remember that nutritional psychiatry is very specialised and should always be overseen by a medical professional. However, for everyday wellness, it does help to understand the basic role of the blood-brain barrier in nutrient bioavailability. It might, for example, guide you in terms of when to serve what to a child who struggles to fall asleep at night. For supper, you might opt for smaller portions of protein and larger portions of carbohydrates that are also rich in tryptophan (like squash or banana). Higher protein portions (e.g., eggs or fermented foods like yoghurt) high in tyrosine (the building block for dopamine) could be a more bioavailable choice for breakfast as dopamine 'upregulates' the nervous systems and is needed for focus. Just remember that balance is key.

Toxins and other Synthetic Chemicals

Toxic chemicals are substances — both synthetic and natural — that will cause harm to human health. They are chemical stressors that can form part of endo-stimulation or exo-stimulation, but we talk about them in this chapter because of their relationship with food.

Not all synthetic chemicals are classified as toxic per se. Still, our bodies are not always able to metabolise synthetic chemicals, making them toxic over a period of time. Apart from absorbing toxins from our environment, we also digest toxins and synthetic chemicals with processed foods or food covered in pesticides.

Organic foods are said typically to have the same amount of nutrients as non-organic foods. Generally speaking, they look and taste more or less the same, too (I would, however, argue that the organic eggs that our two backyard chickens, Koko and Cluck, lay are much tastier and bigger than non-organic eggs, but I might be prejudiced). The real difference lies in the fact that organic food does not contain antibiotics, hormones, or synthetic chemicals and has less of an environmental impact. The negatives of buying organic are that organic food is almost always more expensive and that availability can be an issue. To find a balance, I put the following measures in place for our family, but there are no hard and fast rules:

• I buy organic when my budget allows it and the option is available.

• I have my own organically-raised backyard hens for fresh, organic eggs (the hens were about as much as I could cope with as a working mother with three children, but if you have green fingers and can start your own organic garden, go for it!)

Shortly after my son Néo had his first seizure, I was asked by a naturopathic doctor which kind of folate I took during my pregnancy with Néo. He also wondered if I was one of those people who struggled to metabolise folic acid. It was only years later that I understood the premises of his concerns.

- I soak non-organic fruit and veg in a baking soda solution that gets rid of some of the pesticides. Vinegar and salt make another solution.

- It's a good idea to go organic when it comes to kid-approved-go-tos like ketchup. Just be aware that organic does not necessarily mean low in sugars or salt. It should also be noted that tomatoes can cause problems for some children with food sensitivities.

- With meat products, it's important to look at what the animals were fed and how they were treated. Where possible, I will buy organic or free-range, but unfortunately, it is not always readily available and very expensive. This is not a problem in Vegan diets, but as a family we prefer to include at least some meat and dairy products in our meals.

- If I can pick only a couple of organic items (not including ketchup), I would choose berries, apples, and tomatoes as they have been proven to contain the highest traces of pesticides, as well as milk as it is an affordable staple protein for us (we will discuss the pros and cons of milk in more detail).

We've already touched on the issue of synthetic chemicals in processed foods. But what about foods that are fortified with 'good nutrients'? The problem with fortified foods (as well as many nutritional supplements) is that they do not contain healthy nutrient-synergies - not even when the nutrients used are naturally derived. Synthetic nutrients, unlike their natural versions, are also not always readily metabolised, which can create health issues. The folic acid that most cereals are fortified with and that pregnant women often take in the form of nutritional supplements is but one example. Folic acid is the chemically synthesised form of L-methylfolate (a nutrient critical for the healthy development of a baby, to use one example). However, the process of converting folic acid into L-methylfolate (the most active form of folate) in the body can, in certain people, be slow and inefficient. High levels of unmetabolised folic acid in the bloodstream are linked to various neurological health issues.

According to a study published in the *American Journal of Clinical Nutrition* by C.E. Butterworth and T. Tamura, folic acid may cause neurological injury when given to patients with undiagnosed pernicious anaemia (a condition where folate is not absorbed due to a vitamin B12 deficiency).

Food Packaging

As a working mum of three, I am all for convenience. I think innovative convenience that does not harm the environment or disturb the ESH-Triangle is terrific and needed by modern parents. The problem with convenience is that most of it, like fast food, is provided at the cost of the planet, our health, or both.

I am always so impressed when the suppliers of nutritional supplements, organic products, and water remember not to counter their noble efforts with synthetic plastic packaging. Not only is plastic bad for the environment, but the contents of plastic packaging can be contaminated with plastic particles – even if it is BPA-free. A study published in 2018 by Sherri Mason, a researcher at Penn State Erie, The Behrend College and published in Frontiers in Chemistry, found that plastic contamination in bottled water is rampant. Of the 259 bottled water sold in different countries tested at the time, 93% contained synthetic polymer particles.

Satisfying busy households' need for convenience is important, but it shouldn't be offered at the cost of the planet's health. I recently read an article about an Irish bottling company that has just launched environmentally sensitive, plant-based boxed water products. My advice is to seek out and support innovations like these if you are in the position to do so.

Lastly, consider what you serve food on and with and what you use to clean utensils, water bottles and cutlery.

Nutritional Supplements

Because of soil depletion, our food is not always as nutrient-dense as it should be. Enters your tricky eater, and the need for nutritional support becomes more evident.

The Food Choice Wheel

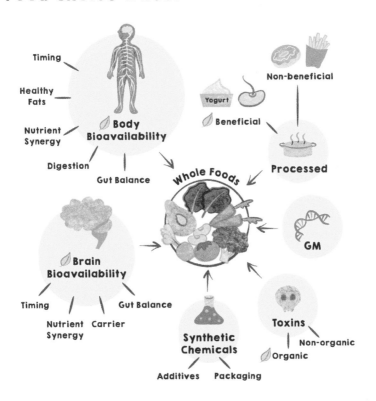

However, the market is cluttered with 'brain-boosting', 'miracle cure' nutritional supplements, and a desperate parent with limited knowledge can feel engulfed. According to the *Child and Maternal Dietary Supplements Market Global Outlook and Forecast 2019-2024*, this market is expected to grow at an annual rate of 10% during this period.

The good news is that the same factors that you would consider when choosing food for your child would apply to nutritional supplements.

Advocating for A Metabolic Evaluation of Children with Developmental or Health Challenges

If you have a child with autism, ADHD, or special needs, you probably already know the major role nutrition plays in support of your child. You might also understand how tricky it can be to get a child with sensory challenges to eat enough - let alone balanced.

Given the importance of nutrition in a child's metabolic (energy system) and therefore overall health, as well as what we know about epigenetics, I believe that every child with developmental or health concerns deserves a metabolic evaluation – regardless of whether the challenges experienced can be linked to a specific genetic fault. The same would apply to a pregnant mother who has certain health or genetic concerns. Specialist-developed, therapeutic diets can make a huge difference in the prevention or support of challenges that any of the three ESH-Triangle pillars may cause.

NUTRITION

Hypothetical Example:

There is a little boy who struggles to focus in school. His teacher says he has anger management issues as well. Concern for him is compounded by the fact that he has recently started to overeat.

It would be easy to jump to any of the following conclusions when reading that narrative: The boy has ADHD. He is suffering from a mood disorder. Or perhaps he has an eating disorder.

What if I told you that instead of three different disorders, there is one reversible metabolic cause for the boy's distress with three symptoms. He is not producing enough of a neurotransmitter called dopamine.

Dopamine is synthesised from an amino acid called tyrosine during brain metabolism. Dopamine plays a crucial role in the concentration, executive functioning and reward networks in the brain. When we enjoy food, we stimulate the release of dopamine.

By overeating, the little boy is trying to make up for the lack of dopamine – he is in a way self-medicating without realising it. The lack of dopamine is also affecting his executive functioning and his ability to focus.

If the little boy was also anxious or struggled to sleep, it might have been worth checking his serotonin levels as well, as this neurotransmitter helps control food cravings.

There are a couple of ways to support the boy – a therapeutic diet is one of them.

The role of nutrition in developmental and health issues experienced by children is undeniable. It is also complex and challenging for parents to navigate. Luckily dietary considerations are becoming increasingly important to clinicians when evaluating and treating their patients.

The purpose of this book is not to diagnose or recommend. Instead, it aims to give you the basic information and tools you need to develop solutions that work for your family and to ask the right questions from the relevant specialised clinicians when you need support.

CHAPTER 10

Nutrients and
their Functions

"Understand the why of nutrition and you will find the how."
– **Alda Smith, Author of** *The Firefly Theory*

Nutrients provide raw fuel for energy, contribute to body structure through chemical building blocks and facilitate or regulates chemical processes in the body once its action potential is activated. This last function of nutrients means that most nutrients also form part of the stimulation pillar in the ESH-Triangle. Given the constant cycle of triangulation within the ESH-Triangle and the dualistic nature of the physical body and energy systems, the overlap between nutrients and stimuli is by now evident. We've already seen how both nutrients and stimulation overlap with DNA in the form of epigenetics, and we will explore this more in Chapter 11 – *Pillar Three: Simulation.*

Our cells require nutrients in much the same way a car requires fuel, oil and water to make it run – the only difference being that a car does not need fuel to build and repair itself.

The eight essential nutrients for humans are:
• Carbohydrates
• Fibre
• Fats (lipids)
• Proteins
• Vitamins
• Minerals
• Water
• Oxygen

1. Fuel for Energy: Carbohydrates, Fats and Oxygen

Carbohydrates are essential nutrients that your body first turns into glucose and then, with the help of oxygen, into ATP (biological currency for energy in the body) via the mitochondria in the cell (see Chapter 5 – *The Mighty Mitochondria* for the critical functions of ATP).

Carbohydrates are also a source of fibre, which we need for the digestion of food. Many fibres, like inulin, act as prebiotics, which 'feed' good gut microbiome or flora needed for digestive and brain health.

The three types of carbohydrates are fibre, starches and sugars. Starches and fibres are called complex carbohydrates and have longer molecule chains with more fibre. Sugars are simple carbohydrates. They have shorter molecules and are quicker to digest.

Examples of food with complex carbohydrates:
• Whole grains and seeds
• Legumes
• Certain vegetables (e.g., potatoes, corn and asparagus)
• Certain fruits (e.g., tomatoes and berries)

Examples of simple carbohydrates:
• Milk
• Fruits
• Refined or processed foods

1.1. Complex Carbohydrates vs Simple Carbohydrates

Generally speaking, most complex carbohydrates are the more nutritious choice as they pack more nutrients (with other functions), are higher in fibre and digest slower. Simple or refined carbohydrates, like sugary foods, do not have much nutritional value other than providing a lot of glucose fast. They don't have fibre and create spikes in blood sugar. However, keep in mind that growing children do not need as much fibre as adults and finding a healthy balance between complex carbohydrates and whole-food simple ones is usually recommended in children.

Even though the body needs a steady supply of carbohydrates, we don't need a lot of it at a time, which is why the 'slow and steady' of complex carbohydrates are preferred. It is important not to deprive a developing child of carbohydrates. When the body is deprived of carbohydrates, it starts tapping into the glycogen stores in the liver. Once the glycogen is depleted, the liver makes ketones from fatty acids and body fat (from there, the term 'keto diet') to keep ATP production going. Although this might be a good way to treat weight issues, children need more body fat for various development processes than adults.

1.2. Too much glucose

Excess glucose in the body is stored in the liver as glycogen or converted into fatty acids stored as fat. Glucose spikes can have a destructive interference with certain antibodies and immune cells, halving their activity for up to five hours following consumption.

Too much insulin, which acts as a glucose gatekeeper to cells, can stimulate pro-inflammatory chemicals called cytokines from human fat cells and other inflammatory molecules that interfere destructively with particular immune cells. This is why carbohydrates are a nutrient to keep an eye on, particularly in children with health or developmental issues.

1.3 Understanding the Glycaemic Index (GI)

The Glycaemic Index (GI) of food shows how quickly a particular food affects your blood glucose level when that food is eaten on its own. That is why complex carbohydrates with a high GI, like particular potatoes, can, like simple carbohydrates, increase blood sugar levels faster than others. The way to manage this is to either stick to complex carbohydrates with medium to low GI's or, if your children like mine love potato, control the portion sizes of complex carbohydrates with higher GI's.

Low GI: 1 – 55   **Medium GI:** 56 – 69   **High GI:** 70 and higher

1.4 Sugars

Sugars fall into two categories – natural (e.g., fructose, honey, or milk sugars) or added sugars (e.g., cane juice or table sugar in processed foods or artificial sugars like aspartame). All sugars essentially do the same thing (provide the raw nutrient for glucose), but a bit of honey on a child's oats is far better than table sugar. The American Heart Association advises that the acceptable amount of 'added sugar' for children under the age of eight is 12 grams per day – that is the equivalent of three teaspoons. A 100ml can of soda contains approximately 10 grams of added sugar.

Even though sugars like agave, xylitol and coconut sugars occur naturally in plants, they still have to go through heavy (in some instances chemical) processing, which moves them away from their 'natural' status.

Artificial sugars like aspartame should also be avoided. Aspartame contains an amino acid called phenylalanine. Too much phenylalanine blocks the production of serotonin (the neurotransmitter that helps us fall asleep and control food cravings). That is also why drinking diet soda to lose weight can be counterproductive.

2. Building Blocks and Cell Energy Stimuli: Proteins and Fats

2.1 Proteins

Proteins are the main ingredient in almost all of our DNA recipes. They provide the physical building blocks for cell structure and energy conduction and expression – the water drops for our rainbows. We also need them to grow and repair cells, turn into antibodies and cell energy stimuli (enzymes, hormones and neurotransmitters), and clot our blood.

Each protein consists of a certain number of amino acids arranged along a 'spine' in a specific sequence. It is estimated that there are more than 80,000 different sequences and therefore proteins in the human body.

There are nine essential and eleven non-essential amino acids. The importance of an amino acid is not determined by whether it is essential or non-essential. Instead, essential amino acids cannot be created by the body. Non-essential amino acids can be metabolised from other nutrients if the gut flora is healthy. This means that unbalanced gut flora can cause deficiencies in non-essential amino acids like tyrosine (the nutrient needed to produce dopamine in the brain).

When a protein source, like eggs, contain all nine essential amino acids, we call it a complete protein. Animal foods are rich in complete proteins. Plant foods are mostly incomplete protein sources. Vegans can combine plant foods to ensure that they get all the essential amino acids they need, but it can be tricky and means that carbohydrate intake will increase. A South American grain called Quinoa is one of the few plant foods that is a complete protein.

Essential Amino Acids	Non-essential Amino Acids
histidine	alanine
isoleucine	arginine*
leucine	asparagine
lysine	aspartic acid
methionine	cysteine*
phenylalanine	glutamine*
threonine	glycine
tryptophan	proline
valine	serine*
	glutamic acid
	tyrosine*

Source: The Metabolic Approach to Cancer

*conditionally essential

2.2. Fats

When we think about fat, we tend to think about obesity and cholesterol. Dietary fats are, however, essential for maintaining good overall health – particularly in developing children.

Fats are lipid molecules (fatty acids) transported through the body's lymphatic system once absorbed. Like carbohydrates, fats also contribute to the creation of ATP in the body's cells.

Fats cannot dissolve in water, making them crucial building blocks for the formation of cell membranes. They are of particular importance to the brain as they act as 'carriers' for neurotransmitters which is vital for signalling in the brain. Fats also help us absorb certain nutrients like vitamins A, D, E, and K and keep cholesterol and blood pressure under control.

There are two types of fats – saturated and unsaturated. Saturated fats are primarily found in animal products. It can become 'solid' and has been demonised as a 'bad fat' that raises cholesterol. However, an increasing amount of research suggests that even though saturated fat can raise both bad and good cholesterol, its overall negative effect is largely determined by sugar.

Unsaturated fats are liquid fats that are seen as healthy. There are two kinds – monounsaturated and polyunsaturated fats. Monounsaturated fats are found in avocados, peanut butter, nuts, and certain seeds. Polyunsaturated fats include Omega 3 and Omega 6, which can be found in hemp seeds, sunflower seeds, flax seeds, fish and algae.

2.3. Omega 3 and Omega 6

Not all Omega 3 fats are the same. The four most important ones are DHA, DPA, EPA and ALA.

DHA, DPA and EPA form a long-chain molecule (n-3 LC-PUFA) and

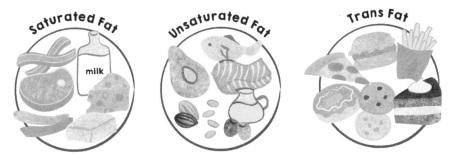

are mainly found in fatty fish and algae. n-3 LC-PUFA can prevent mental health issues, cardiovascular disease, cancer as well as inflammatory diseases.

ALA, which is mostly found in plant foods, has to be metabolised into EPA or DHA for the body to use it for something other than energy. Recent research suggests this conversion process to be inefficient for the amount of n-3LC-PUFA required by the human body.

Omega 6, mainly found in plant foods (vegetable oils), also has certain health benefits, such as lowering bad cholesterol. Some research advocates that this fat can be pro-inflammatory, which is why many clinicians indicate that they are consumed in moderation if, for example, a gut imbalance is suspected.

2.4 Trans Fats

Trans fats are the fats to avoid. Apart from a minimal amount in some animal products, trans fats do not really exist in nature. They are unsaturated fats (vegetable oils) that are changed through processing.

3. Cell Energy Stimuli, Soldiers and Cleaners: Vitamins and Minerals

Vitamins are organic molecules found in living organisms. Minerals are inorganic molecules that are absorbed by organisms through the water and ground. Both are used by the body to 'stimulate' other nutrients like proteins into a particular shape and function.

Different vitamins and minerals stimulate different functions. These functions determine a nutrient's role in the body. This is why all nutrients, including vitamins and minerals, actually form part of the stimulation pillar once absorbed and 'activated'.

3.1 The Roles of Vitamins and Minerals

The roles of vitamins and minerals vary, but they can be summarised as follows:
- To create nutrient synergy and bioavailability for better absorption.
- To support the production or activation of cell energy stimulants (including signalling molecules like hormones or neurotransmitters and catalysts like enzymes).
- To facilitate healthy cell division, growth and repair.
- To prevent cell or DNA damage by stimulating and controlling the production of antibodies and inflammation for fighting germs and irritants.
- To prevent cell or DNA damage by protecting against or removing free radicals or unwanted chemicals.

3.2. Phytonutrients

Phytonutrients are medically active compounds found in plants that are neither vitamin nor mineral, for example, carotenoids, betaine, choline, catechins, curcuminoids and saponins.

Phytonutrients are believed to work with vitamins and minerals to prevent and repair DNA and cell damage by protecting the body against pathogens, toxins, free radicals and inflammation. Foods rich in phytonutrients include Brussels sprouts, broccoli, red bell peppers, paprika, green tea, beetroot, carrots, turmeric and garlic.

Vitamin	Function	Food Examples
A	Growth	Kale + Eggs + Carrots
B1 (Thiamine)	Energy + Synergy	Eggs + Milk + Legumes
B2 (Riboflavin)	Energy	Spinach + Mushrooms
B3 (Niacin)	Energy + Guard + Clean	Chicken + Avocado + Fish
B6 (Pyridoxine)	Energy + Guard + Clean + Synergy	Fish + Kale + Bananas
B7 (Biotin)	Guard	Mushrooms + Seaweed + Milk
L-Methylfolate	Energy + Growth + Synergy	Spinach + Asparagus + Liver
B12	Energy + Growth + Synergy	Liver + Eggs + Mushrooms
C	Guard + Clean	Strawberries + Brussels Sprouts + Brocolli

NUTRITION

Vitamin	Function	Food Examples
D	Guard + Synergy	Algae + Mushrooms + Red meat
E	Guard + Clean + Synergy	Olive Oil + Sunflower Seeds + Pumkin
K	Energy	Kale + Turnip + Seaweed

Minerals	Function	Food examples
Calcium	Growth + Energy	Brocolli + Milk + Spinach
Magnesium	Energy	Brocolli + Algae + Beetroot
Iron	Energy	Red Meat + Beans + Beetroot
Copper	Synergy	Meat + Algae
Zinc	Energy + Guard	Meat + Peas

4. Water and Oxygen

Both water and oxygen are essential for life. The human body consists of approximately 64% of water, mostly found in the cell cytoplasm. Not only does it therefore have structural purposes, but it is also the carrier for nutrients, including oxygen to the cells, as well as toxins being flushed from the body. This is why a glass of water before school and before bedtime (if bedwetting is not a problem) is beneficial to children.

Water keeps our eyes, noses and mouths moist and protects our organs. If you prefer bottled water, it is important to note the packaging, as mentioned earlier. Tap water should be filtered if possible.

Without oxygen, we can't produce ATP, and the body will not have the energy it needs to function. That is why a bit of exercise or fresh air can improve focus and other brain functions.

It has been postulated that children with severe neurological challenges may benefit from oxygen therapy, but it requires expert regulation, as too much oxygen can be damaging and even deadly. Plants that purify the air and increase oxygen levels in bedrooms and classrooms are a safer everyday alternative.

NUTRITION

5. Food Allergies and Sensitivities

Allergies and sensitivities will be discussed in more detail in Chapter 13 – *The Immune System* as they are inappropriate immune responses. We will, however, touch on two food sensitivities that seem to plague our children: lactose and gluten intolerance.

5.1 Lactose (and Casein)

Milk is a 'complete protein,' which makes it an affordable protein staple for many families. Milk, however, contains a lot of milk sugar called lactose, which is often blamed for lactose intolerance in children.

People who are lactose intolerant do not have enough effective lactase, which is an enzyme needed to metabolise milk sugar. What most parents do not know, however, is that when fat is removed from milk, the sugar (lactose) content increases. This is important because if switching from low fat to whole milk is not a possible compromise for some children with less severe lactose sensitivities, it is, according to a growing group of nutritional researchers, at the very least a healthier option due to the balance of fat to sugar to protein (remember whole milk is a whole-food).

It might also help to know that lactose is broken down into simpler sugars during fermentation, which means that some lactose-intolerant children may be okay with fermented dairies like yoghurt or kefir.

We might also erroneously be putting all the milk intolerance blame on the lactose in it. As mentioned before, milk is a good complete protein source. A protein called casein accounts for approximately 80% of the protein in milk. About 30% of this is beta-casein. There are thirteen kinds of beta-caseins, but the two to take note of are A1 and A2. Over 8,000 years ago, cow milk only contained A2-caseins. Today most of the milk we buy from the store has only A1-casein or a combination of the two.

According to an article in *Medical News Today*, the molecule structure of the A2 protein is more comparable to those in human breast milk, goats and sheep, than that of the A1 protein. Some researchers believe that it is, in fact, A1 proteins that are responsible for many of the symptoms usually blamed on lactose.

If you are a milk-drinking family and you suspect dairy sensitivities, it might be worth talking to your doctor about trying organic, whole A2 milk first before eliminating it. In severe milk allergies, it might also be beneficial to determine if lactose or A1 protein is the culprit.

5.2 Gluten

Gluten is a seed-storage protein found in grains like wheat, barley, rye and triticale that provides no essential nutrients. Some people have an immune reaction (inflammation) in their small intestines when eating gluten.

When this happens, the lining of the small intestine can be damaged, which interferes with the absorption of nutrients.

The digestive system has to work hard to break down gluten, so removing gluten from a diet can often lead to automatic energy increases.

Sprouted grain flours and sourdough bread are all ways to assist with the breakdown of gluten to remove some of the stress it can cause the digestive system.

NUTRITION

A FINAL NOTE OF ENCOURAGEMENT FROM THE AUTHOR

> "Simple can be harder than complex: You have to work hard to get your thinking clean to make it simple. But it's worth it in the end because once you get there, you can move mountains."
>
> **– Steve Jobs**

To help you come to a place of simplicity, I've walked you through some pretty complex science. You might even feel a bit overwhelmed. Unless you are a doctor or researcher, you don't have to remember every single detail. A stereogram is not about the individual grains but the bigger picture. As parents, we want to understand, love and support our children – not be their clinicians.

With these last chapters, it might feel like it gets even more complex before it becomes simpler. This note is to reassure you that the bigger picture is on its way! We might not understand or change everything we are faced with in our children's health and development, but we will understand or change nothing if it is not faced. We've faced child development and health from the cell up – it's almost time to see what we can influence and how we can influence it.

STIMULATION

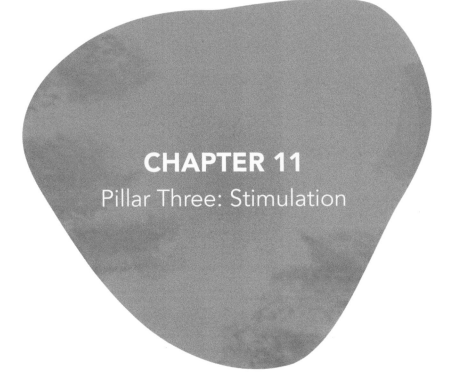

CHAPTER 11
Pillar Three: Stimulation

"A spark is a little thing, yet it may kindle the world."
— **Martin Farquhar Tupper, Author of** *Proverbial Philosophy*

Finally! The last pillar in the ESH-Triangle and arguably the most important one. We've come full circle on *The Firefly Theory*'s quantum-mechanical-chemical perspective on the energy system. This is where it all begins and ends.

The Spark of Life

The human body exists of matter (molecules and cells) that vibrates at certain frequencies – such frequencies determine the shape and function potential of the molecules and cells. For molecules to arrange themselves so that life can be expressed through them and for function potential to be sparked into a working energy system (life), something needs to stimulate and direct the molecules and cells. DNA and nutrients alone will not make a cell function or grow – it needs stimulation. This is the spark of life.

Think of a plant seed. It is not dead, but it is not alive either. It is resting in potential. Without the sun, water and nutrients stimulating it, its energy won't be harnessed for a plant to grow. Add the right stimuli, and the resting potential will be activated into a living plant.

STIMULATION

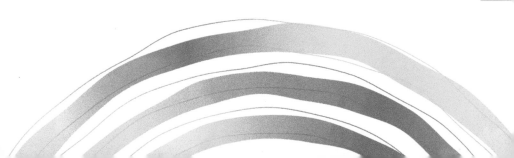

Stimulation and Controls

Stimulation is the action of exciting something into shape and/or function and destruction by letting the stimulus's energy vibrations interfere with its target's energy vibrations. Four stimulus controls determine the constructive and destructive effects of stimulation:

- Frequency (wave)
- Duration
- Intensity
- Recurrence (how often)

Stimulation can be chemical (nutrients), mechanical (sound vibrations), or 'holographic' (our thoughts and emotions) in nature. Depending on the stimulus controls and objective, stimuli can positively or negatively affect the energy system. They can also be neutral. A negative stimulus is called a 'stressor.' For example, the sun emits light at lower frequencies (near-infrared), which with certain durations and recurrences can have healing effects as it supports the last step in the cell respiration process discussed earlier. It also emits light at higher frequencies (ultraviolet) that can damage humans but is useful in sterilising medical equipment.

Certain synthetic chemicals used in foods are, in theory, harmless to humans. However, over time they can become harmful. Coldwater swimming has many health benefits, but depending on the controls, low temperatures for extended periods can also cause hypothermia.

In *The Firefly Theory* context, stimulation can come from outside the body (exo) or inside the body (endo) itself.

Exo-Stimulation

The exo-stimulation system refers to our environment. A developing child needs different forms of stimulation from outside the body. In *Disconnected Kids*, Dr Robert Melillo illustrates the importance of external stimulation for the developing child by highlighting a case study of orphanages in Romania in which abandoned babies, left in cribs without any interaction, experienced underdeveloped brains almost to the point of intellectual disability.

Our senses are the gatekeepers that allow exo-stimuli (often referred to as 'sensory input') to reach our brain and other cells. These include our eyes, ears, noses, skin and mouths (linked to our digestive system). It is safe to say that medicine and therapy have their roots in exo-stimuli.

Mechanical exo-stimuli include:
- Sound vibration
- Light vibration
- Touch or pressure
- Physical exercise and movement in relation to space and gravity
- Sleep (crosses over with endo-stimuli)
- Primitive reflexes (crosses over with endo-stimuli)
- Electromagnetic vibration
- Temperature
- Pathogens
- Targeted therapies that utilise any of the above (e.g., occupational therapy, reflexology and light therapy)

Chemical exo-stimuli include:
- Food, oxygen and water (nutrients)
- Synthetic chemicals
- Toxins
- Odour
- Taste
- Targeted therapies that use any of the above (e.g., nutritional therapy, aromatherapy and medication)

Quantum exo-stimuli include:
- Positive and negative experiences within our environment (e.g., love, trauma, etc.)
- Intellectual exercises (e.g., reading and learning)
- Targeted therapies that utilise any of the above (e.g., psychotherapy)

STIMULATION

Mechanical Exo-Stimuli

Sound
Vibration

Light

Touch

Physical
Exercise

Temperature

Primitive
Reflexes

Sleep

Pathogens

Electromagnetic
Vibration

Targeted
Therapies

Chemical Exo-Stimuli

Nutrients

Synthetic
Chemicals

Toxins

Odour

Taste

Targeted
Therapies

Quantum Exo-Stimuli

Positive &
Negative
Experiences

Intellectual
Exercises

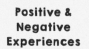
Targeted
Therapies

Chemical Endo-Stimuli

Neurotransmitters　　　**ATP**　　　**Mitochondrial Signalling**　　　**Hormones**

Enzymes　　　**Nutrients**　　　**Adrenaline**　　　**Antibodies**

Platelet-Derived Growth Factors　　　**Inflammatory Chemicals**　　　**Antioxidants**　　　**Targeted Therapies**

Mechanical Endo-Stimuli

Electrical Pulses in Neurons　　　**Heartbeat**

Pathogens　　　**Human Cells**

Quantum Endo-Stimuli

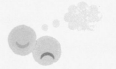

Perceptions, Emotions, Thoughts and Memories

Endo-Stimulation

The body's endo-stimulation systems consist of our energy system and all our physical body systems, of which the nervous and the immune systems are probably the most important for purposes of this book.

Mechanical endo-stimuli include:
- Electrical pulses produced in neurons
- Heartbeat
- Pathogens (e.g. gut flora)
- Cells (structural integrity of the ESH-Prism)

Chemical endo-stimuli include:
- Neurotransmitters
- ATP
- Mitochondrial signalling
- Hormones

- Enzymes
- Nutrients
- Adrenaline
- Antibodies
- Platelet-derived growth factors (PDGF)
- Inflammatory chemicals
- Antioxidants

Quantum endo-stimuli include:
- Positive and negative thoughts, perceptions and emotions

An Accumulative Effect

When we looked at gut balance in Chapter 8 – *The Chapter before Nutrition*, we saw how any stimulation can have a positive or negative accumulative effect. Bacterial overgrowth does not only affect how nutrients are absorbed, but it actually has a chain reaction throughout the body. The same is true for therapeutic stimulation.

An exo-stimulus example is lavender – it can have a calming effect, contributing to better sleep. Good sleep helps the brain to repair and grow, which has a positive effect on our immune system and many other functions.

Therapeutic stimuli should be applied with this in mind. A layered strategy is always more effective.

Mind over Matter

Dr Patrick Nemechek, author of *The Nemechek Protocol for Autism and Development Disorders*, describes the underlying cause of most diseases as 'the failure of our brains that sets into motion the failure of our bodies.' He is right – following the instructions of its DNA (which itself is affected by stimulation), the brain 'translates' all exo-stimuli into an integrated endo-stimuli-driven metabolic response, called life. The brain is the biggest source of stimuli within the body or the ESH-Triangle. These include electrical signals, neurotransmitters, thoughts, perceptions and emotions. If the brain does not function, there is nothing to direct the molecules in the body. Without stimulation or interference, they will remain at resting potential, the body or endo-stimulation systems can't function, and the organic matter of the body will eventually break down.

Let's think of Dr George Gonzalez's metaphor of life being like a rainbow projected through water. It becomes easier to see how – with the brain and nervous system at the tip – the body acts as an ESH-Prism with the ESH-Triangle as its trusty foundation. Much like a rainbow is created when a light source hits a prism, the brain and nervous system translate the exo-stimuli it receives through the senses into endo-stimuli, which, with the help of the other two ESH-pillars, express the rainbow of life.

Structurally, the prism should be intact for the energy system to be expressed through (a tethered spinal cord, for example, can't conduct energy as it should). We should never overlook structural causes of energy system failure, but as the biggest source of stimuli within the body, the brain almost always plays a role and most if not all disease or dysfunction is accumulative in nature.

STIMULATION

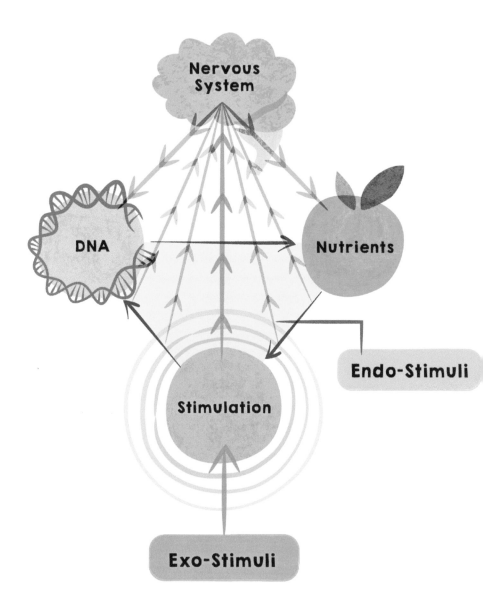

ESH-Triangle Prism

Stimuli and the Unbalanced Brain

It is important to understand that as much as the exo- and endo-stimuli (or the lack thereof) affect the body, it also affects the brain that acts as the bridge between them. Like Dr Nemechek, one could argue that both the health and the dysfunction of the energy system and the body it is expressed through, start in the brain. Imbalances within the nervous system are necessary to create the tension needed for triangulation within the energy system, but if the energy system is consistently out of balance in the brain, it will be out of balance in the body, which can lead to dysfunction.

When the brain is out of balance, it can struggle to cope with the stimuli from outside and even inside the body. Once this happens, even neutral stimuli (like a label in the back of a shirt) can become stressors. A child constantly experiencing neutral stimuli as stressors may be described as sensory defensive or 'stimuli defensive'. The opposite is also true. An unbalanced brain might find regular stimuli 'too weak' and become 'sensory seeking' or 'stimuli seeking'. A child running into things on purpose or chewing things for extra feedback is often driven by a sensory seeking nervous system. The same is true if the brain is not producing enough of a certain endo-stimulus like the neurotransmitter dopamine. When this happens, it might 'seek' the interference of this stimulus by 'instructing' the child to overeat.

Because different neurons fire at different frequencies, the brain may also try to find stimuli frequencies that activate certain neurons or de-activate others when it feels out of balance in a particular situation. Think of a child making low humming sounds when trying to feel calm or the white noise sounds that help babies sleep.

STIMULATION

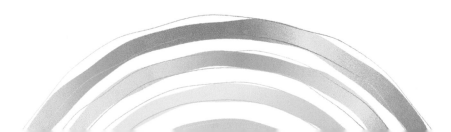

When the brain tries to have a balanced experience of stimuli or sensory input, we say it 'regulates'. Up-regulation is when more of a specific kind of stimuli interference is employed. Down-regulation is when the interference of certain stimuli is decreased, or excess energy from it is released. A meltdown can be compared to a nervous system 'burp' to expel energy the body can't use in a helpful way.

All of us engage in self-regulatory behaviour like whistling, humming or even nail biting to support our brains in its effort to find balance. Self-regulatory repetitive behaviours in children with neurological challenges, called stimming, are no different in their cause. It might just take on a more a-typical form like hair pulling or hand flapping. On the face of it, there is nothing wrong with self-regulatory behaviour. It is when it becomes destructive or affects a child's ability to function that alternatives need to be looked at.

An unbalanced brain might also struggle to integrate the exo-stimuli into a cohesive response. If persistent, this is referred to as sensory integrational challenges.

The Nervous and Immune Systems

In Chapter 10 – *Nutrients and their Functions*, we saw that nutrients facilitate or regulate chemical processes in the body and that nutrients and stimulation overlap. As the biggest source of stimulation inside the body, the brain works closely with its second-in-command – the gut (also known as the 'second brain') – which is why we will often hear about the importance of gut-brain health. Although the gut-brain symbiosis is very important, the brain not only relies on the gut, but on all the other body or endo-stimulation systems it works so hard to direct. For example, for the brain to direct the other endo-systems, it still needs oxygen from the respiratory and cardiovascular systems. Like with the pillars in the ESH-Triangle, it is very much a 'chicken and egg' situation.

The purpose of *The Firefly Theory* is to provide parenting, educational and healthcare communities with a universal model for optimal nervous system development and immune priming in children. The aim is also to furnish you with a 'blueprint' to develop your own functional, integrated and collaborative strategy for the prevention and counter of adverse developmental and health events before and after birth. It is for this reason and for reasons explained through the ESH-Triangle Prism that *The Firefly Theory's* regulation and modulation methods are rooted in the nervous system (including the brain), together with our immune system (of which 75-85% consists of the digestive system – see Chapter 8 – *The Chapter Before Nutrition*). We will explore these two systems in more detail over the next two chapters.

STIMULATION

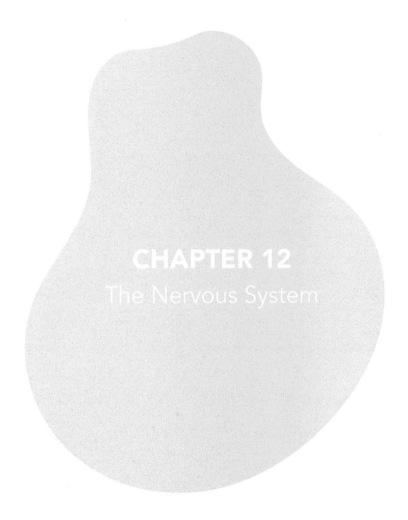

CHAPTER 12
The Nervous System

> "In many ways, the nervous system works like a computer. It's, therefore,
> time we became better programmers."
> **– Alda Smith, Author of** *The Firefly Theory*

Stimulation and the Nervous System

The nervous system is divided into two dualistic systems – the central nervous system (CNS) and the peripheral nervous system (PNS). The central system consists of your brain and spinal cord, whereas your peripheral nervous system comprises a network of nerves branching out from the spinal cord.

The CNS receives and integrates all the stimuli the PNS collects from the somatic sensory system (senses) and visceral sensory system (organs and other body systems) into a cohesive endo- and exo-response. Such responses can be both conscious (voluntary) or unconscious (involuntary). The voluntary responses are communicated via the somatic motor system and the involuntary stimuli via the autonomic nervous system. The brain does the translation and integration, while the spinal cord acts as a two-way highway between the brain and the PNS – one lane for input stimuli (chemical and electrical messages going to the brain) and the other for output (instructional chemical and electrical messages going from the brain to the rest of the body).

STIMULATION

Nervous Tissue

Nervous tissue is densely packed with cells. When we think of nerve cells, we think of neurons. The neurons respond to stimuli and transmit electrical signals and chemical stimuli called neurotransmitters. Neurons are not all the same – they come in different sizes and have specialised functions. They do, however, have the following in common:

• they are some of the longest-lived cells in the body.
• they cannot be replaced.
• they are energy-hungry and need a steady supply of glucose and oxygen for ATP production.

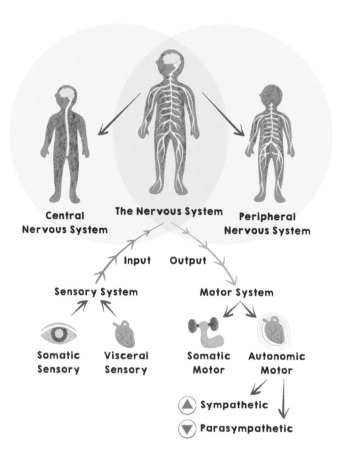

Neurons all have the same structure, which consists of a cell body (with a nucleus, DNA, mitochondria and other organelles), the dendrites (stimuli receivers) and a long extension called the axon (stimuli sender). Some axons can run from the brain all the way down the CNS to the feet.

Sensory neurons (mostly unipolar) sends stimuli or signals from the sensory nervous system to the brain. Motor neurons (mostly multipolar) send stimuli away from the nervous system to the rest of the body. Interneurons (also mostly multipolar) in the CNS connect the sensory and motor neurons.

Neurons are surrounded and protected by glial cells. There are different types of glial cells. Not only are they the glue holding the neurons together, but as seen in Chapter 8 – *The Chapter Before Nutrition*, they are also involved in neuron repair and pruning – a function that is adversely affected by a 'leaky gut.' They also anchor neurons to the blood supply in the brain, forming part of the blood-brain barrier and the immune system.

Electrical Signals, Neurotransmitters, Synapses and Neural Pathways

The nervous system's strength lies in the connection of neurons. Without it, stimuli can't be passed along, and the neurons will stay in resting potential. The meeting point between a neuron's axon and another neuron's dendrites is called a synapse. There are electrical synapses for fast and direct communication (e.g., communication with the heart) and chemical synapses for selected, slower and more controlled communication.

When a neuron is stimulated, it sends an electrical message to the end of its axon, picked up by the next neuron's dendrites. The electrical message can either be sent directly through electrical synapses

STIMULATION

for fast communication or turned into chemical messages called neurotransmitters that cross the synaptic cleft, a small gap between the synapses. Depending on the kind of neurotransmitter, it can either excite the next neuron to create a new charge or inhibit the neuron (like serotonin that inhibits neurons for sleep). After the neurotransmitters have delivered their message, they either degrade or are taken back up by the neuron that sent them. It is this mechanism that a lot of chemical drugs use for therapeutic effects – both inhibitory and excitatory.

New experiences will stimulate certain neurons to signal other neurons, forming a network. The strength of such a network will be determined by the frequency (wave), duration, intensity and recurrence (how often) of its stimulation.

The Brain Regions

The brain is the most complex organ. It is the control centre for the whole body, and trillions of electrical and chemical pulses pass along its complex network every second.

The largest structure in the brain, called the cerebrum, controls higher brain functions such as memory, executive functioning, speech and vision. The outer layer of the cerebrum is called the cortex. The cerebrum has a left hemisphere and a right hemisphere that consist of different regions with different specialised functions:
- Frontal cortex (also known as the 'rational brain') – executive functioning, planning, problem-solving, etc.
- Motor area – movement
- Sensory area – processes exo-stimuli received from our senses
- Visual area – processes information from the eyes
- Temporal lobes – emotions, memory, hearing and speech

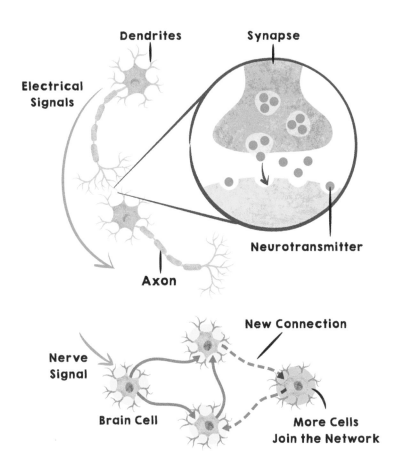

The left and right hemispheres communicate with each other via a thick bundle of nerve fibres.

Below the cerebrum, towards the back of the brain, lies the cerebellum, which controls balance and co-ordination. It is the co-ordinator of the brain and supports smooth and balanced activity.

Underneath the frontal cortex lies a subcortical complex called the limbic system, which is also home to what is known as our 'emotional brain' and our 'reptilian brain.' This part of our brain forms part of our autonomic nervous system and is responsible for emotions and urges and 'involuntary' body systems like the cardiovascular system.

The different areas of the brain and the two hemispheres have to work together in an integrated manner. Stimuli and DNA can cause any of these areas to get out of balance, e.g., one area of the brain might become stronger than the other. When this happens, the energy system becomes unbalanced, and the brain does not have the synergy it needs for optimal development and health.

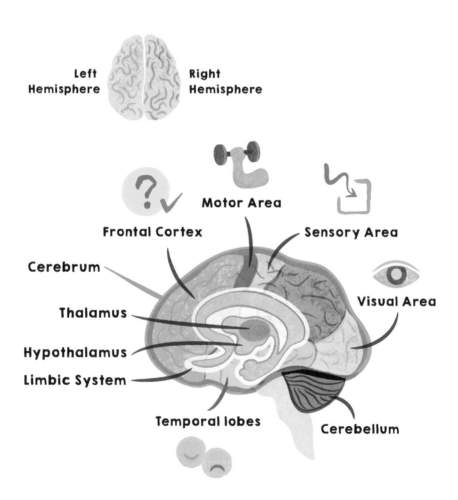

The Autonomic Nervous System

When referring to self-control, we refer to a 'higher' function of the cortex and the frontal cortex specifically. This has wrongly created the impression that our cortex (our rational brain) is more powerful than the limbic system (our irrational or impulse brain). As described by Dr Stuart Shanker in his book, *Self-Reg*, a more helpful viewpoint is that of the autonomic nervous system (including the limbic system) as the foundation that the cortex rests on. This idea is cemented by the fact that the frontal cortex is only fully developed by the age of 25.

As the foundation of our nervous system, the autonomic nervous system plays a vital role in a child's development and wellness. If the autonomic nervous system is 'shaky,' the frontal cortex will show some 'cracks.' The power of rational thinking and action is far outweighed by a highly stressed autonomic nervous system. Think of a child having a melt-down. It would be a mistake to try and reason with someone whose autonomic nervous system is in overdrive. Only once the balance is restored, the reasonable frontal cortex might be engaged.

The hypothalamus, which lies within the limbic system, is viewed as the master of our involuntary endo-stimuli systems. It plays a critical role in the immune system, body temperature, hunger, heart rate, breathing, endocrine system (hormones), sleep, hearing and emotional cues. These functions are tied to our brain and body's most primitive responses to stimulation and require continuous regulation to achieve balance. If it's cold outside, the body will heat up. If it's warm, the sweat glands will open up. The sympathetic and parasympathetic nervous systems regulate the arousal state in the autonomic nervous system. The sympathetic system activates body systems (upregulates) and is mainly controlled by the splanchnic nerves, and the parasympathetic nervous system calms the body systems down (downregulates) and is controlled by the vagus nerve.

STIMULATION

Another area in the limbic system worth mentioning is the thalamus. It processes and passes on all the exo-stimuli received by the senses. Our sense of smell is, for example, processed here. The fact that the thalamus is so close to the hypothalamus (where emotions are triggered) can partially explain why we have such strong emotional connections to smells and songs or sounds. As seen earlier in Chapter 9 – *Pillar Two: Nutrition*, an underdeveloped sense of smell is often present in tricky eaters, who often also have other neurological challenges, which again illustrates the cascading effect of imbalances in the energy and central nervous systems.

An example of an imbalance in the autonomic nervous system is when the body is stuck in 'high alert mode,' i.e., the sympathetic nervous system keeps overriding the parasympathetic nervous system. If something is perceived as a threat, the sympathetic side of the nervous system will trigger neuro-chemicals, like adrenaline, required to create a 'fight-or-flight' response. Chemicals like adrenaline and cortisol stimulate energy production in the major muscles. Endorphins are released, pain tolerance increases and energy is directed away from functions that are viewed as non-essential in the immediate context of the 'threat'. Although this is an essential function for survival, it becomes problematic when the parasympathetic nervous system fails to counter the reactions. Dr Shanker explains that when this happens, essential functions, like the immune system, the frontal cortex function, sleep and even hearing, that were viewed as non-essential in the moment, break down. These cascading effects of an imbalance in the autonomic nervous system can have many developmental and health consequences for children. As seen in Chapter 11 – *Pillar Three: Stimulation*, an imbalance can also result in an inability to cope with stimuli from outside and even inside the body. Even neutral stimuli can become stressors, and the entire central nervous system can become overloaded and unable to cope. Ways to downregulate the autonomic nervous system include stressor removal, gut balancing, as well as vagus nerve priming (e.g., chiropractic alignment) and stimulation (e.g., singing, yawing, electrotherapy and certain medications).

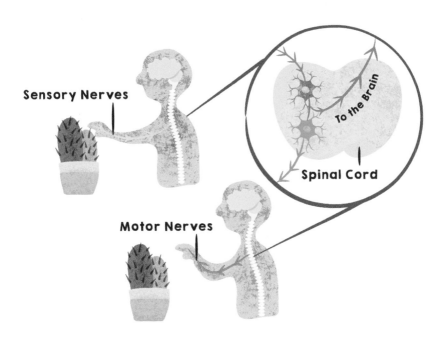

Sensory Nerves

Motor Nerves

To the Brain

Spinal Cord

Reflex Arc Pathway

Reflexes

Reflexes are automatic responses to internal and external stimuli. To save time in certain situations, the stimuli bypass the brain's interpretation and go directly from the sensory nerves to the motor nerves. This is made possible by something called a reflex arc, which acts as an intersection between the sensory nervous system, the motor nervous system and the central nervous system. Reflexes are essential because they provide protective responses to maintain a state of balance. If you burn your finger, the stimulus will cross the reflex arc, activating an immediate reflex response within the motor nerves to pull away and simultaneously sending a pain signal to the brain. Babies are born with what is called primitive reflexes, which also require no thought. These reflexes, like rooting, sucking and startle reflexes, help the baby during birth and the first weeks of life. As the nervous system matures, primitive reflexes are no longer needed, and the brain starts to inhibit them. When these primitive reflexes are not brought under control, they can interfere with other developmental phases and processes. When this happens, they become a source of unwelcome 'noise.'

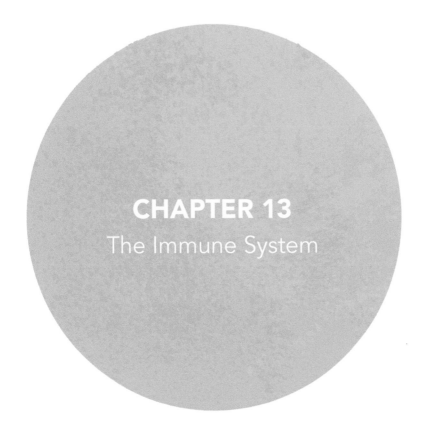

CHAPTER 13
The Immune System

> "Sickness and dysfunction can be the result of an overactive or a compromised immune system. The idea of simply 'boosting' the immune system is, therefore, slightly flawed. We should instead aim to balance and prime."
> **– Alda Smith, Author of** *The Firefly Theory*

The Innate and Adaptive Immune System

Our immune systems are made up of different cells, soluble and organs, such as the skin and digestive tract. It is the body's collective defence measures against pathogens, including bacteria, viruses, fungi and parasites – all of which stimulate the body's energy system in unhelpful ways.

Babies are born with an innate immune system. As they grow, they are exposed to more and more pathogens either by naturally encountering them or being vaccinated, and so, the adaptive immune system develops. Breastfeeding, to a certain extent, lets a newborn benefit from the mother's adaptive immune system.

Physical and Chemical Barriers

Skin and membranes provide physical barriers against germs and other body invaders. Fluids like tears, mucus and saliva provide chemical resistance against bacteria that can cause physical damage to body tissue and chemical viruses that can take control of the body's cells.

Gut Flora

As seen in Chapter 8 – *The Chapter Before Nutrition*, the gut makes up 75-85% of the immune system. Helpful bacteria in our gut support the

STIMULATION

immune system by contributing to the breakdown and absorption of all nutrients needed by the immune system while making certain toxins, poisons, dangerous bacteria and viruses stay away. Although antibiotics kill bacteria, they can also kill the 'good' bacteria in the gut.

The Lymphatic System

The lymphatic system collects and drains away excess fluid that has passed from the blood. Consisting of the spleen, tonsils and lymph nodes, it also carries cells that can help with the fight against infection by blocking pathogens from spreading around the body.

A paediatrician once explained that he did not want to remove Néo's chronically infected tonsils too soon because, in very young babies, tonsils could help keep pathogens out of the lungs where they can wreak even more havoc.

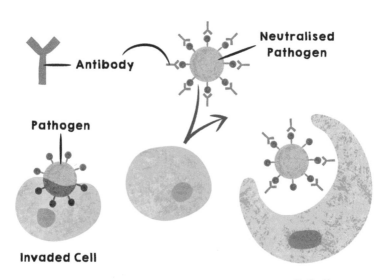

White Blood Cells and Antibodies

When the first lines of defence are crossed, the immune system still has an army of special white blood cells that can kill viruses and bacteria by eating them or neutralising them with chemicals. Most white blood cells were once stem cells that came from the bone marrow tissue. There are different kinds of white blood cells, but the two main ones are B-cells and T-cells. The difference between B-cells and T-cells is that the first neutralise the pathogens and the second kill cells already infected by the pathogen. T-cells also receive their finishing touches in the thymus gland, which sits behind the sternum between your lungs (from there, the 'T').

Once a B-cell has killed a virus or a bacteria, it multiplies and releases a chemical protein called antibodies specific to the enemy killed. Antibodies attach themselves to the invaders to flag them as enemies for the white blood cells to eat. Antibodies can also create a barrier around the invader so that it can't attach to other cells, neutralising it.

Microglia are a small type of glial cells in the brain. Because the brain is separated from the rest of the body by the blood-brain barrier, microglia act as the brain's own immune system. Microglia get rid of pathogens and toxins. They cause inflammation as part of the healing process but can become overactive when energy imbalances, e.g., gut health issues, occur.

Inflammation and Fever

Inflammation is a normal immune system response to fight infection or repair tissue damage. When tissue in the body is damaged or stressed, inflammatory chemicals like cytokines and histamines are released. These chemicals increase blood flow and signal white blood cells to fight infection. Inflammation can lead to redness, heat and pain.

STIMULATION

Inflammation is partly regulated by the autonomic nervous system, with the sympathetic nervous system as the 'activator.' If pro-inflammatory proteins become too abundant and aggressive, they can start to damage healthy organs and tissue in an autoimmune response. This can lead to or fuel inflammatory autoimmune diseases such as cardiovascular disease, certain types of diabetes, neurological conditions, developmental delays and certain mood and behavioural disorders.

When discussing COVID-19 in a 2020 interview, Prof Patrick Bouic, an Immunology Professor at the University of Stellenbosch, said that some research would suggest that it is this kind of cytokine storm induced by the COVID-19 virus that ultimately does more damage than the virus itself, which is why people suffering from inflammatory diseases, such as asthma, cardiovascular diseases or autoimmune diseases were considered more vulnerable.

Beyond its function in calcium balance, vitamin D has recently been found to play an essential role in the modulation of inflammation, which is one reason it is encouraged in the wake of the COVID-19 pandemic. Regulating glucose levels can also be a natural way to control inflammation, as insulin spikes can trigger pro-inflammatory chemicals.

Fevers can be a system-wide sign of inflammation that raises the body temperature to stimulate an immune response. The body can elevate the temperature to fight infection as well. High temperatures and levels of pro-inflammatory can lower the seizure threshold in the brain, which is why some children get febrile seizures when they have a fever.

Sensitivities and Allergies

Histamines are signalling molecules that stimulate various important functions, like the increase of stomach acids. Like cytokines, it also helps the B-cells in fighting invaders. Similar to how cytokine storms can make people very sick, too many histamines can cause allergies like hay fever, skin allergy and food allergy. An allergic reaction is when the immune system treats non-threatening substances as invaders. When this happens, a cascading array of symptoms can occur, from swelling, tearing, struggling to breathe to anaphylaxis.

A food allergy is an overreaction to a harmless food protein. Even though there is a lot to be learned about allergies in general, more and more research suggests that babies are not born with it in general. Instead, allergies develop as the baby's immune system matures, which means genetics, gut health, and immune system regulation (or the lack thereof) all play a role. Interestingly, avoiding certain foods in early infancy can also increase the risks of allergies to those foods, making a case for the controlled introduction of allergens as a form of 'allergy immunisation' whereby the immune system can be trained to recognise food proteins as harmless.

Food sensitivities are not the same as allergies in that they do not produce physical, identifiable allergic reactions. According to Dr Robert Melillo, author of *Disconnected Kids*, food sensitivities instead produce an inflammatory response that results in subtle mental and behavioural symptoms from bed wetting to meltdowns.

Antioxidants

Antioxidants protect cells and tissue from damage by removing free radicals and toxins from the body. It is even said to, in some instances, repair cell damage. This, in turn, improves various immune responses in the body, which is why people are encouraged to stock up on antioxidants during flu season. Examples of nutrients that act as antioxidants are Vitamin C and E.

STIMULATION

CHAPTER 14
Changing the Course
of your Child's Health
and Development

> "The human race will never be stronger than its next generation."
> – **Alda Smith, Author of** *The Firefly Theory*

Regulation can be defined as the action of balancing. As seen earlier, up-regulation is when more of a specific kind of stimulus interference is employed. Down-regulation is when the interference of certain stimuli is decreased, or excess energy from it is released. In therapy, regulation refers to the child's ability to increase or decrease overall arousal through stimulation to function optimally.

Modulation can be defined as the interventions or adjustments made to help achieve regulation or a balanced state.

Throughout this book, we have seen how DNA, nutrients and stimulation (the ESH-Triangle) form the foundation of balance within the energy system. In this final chapter, you will be given a framework called the *ESH-Prism Regulation and Modulation Method* to guide you in supporting your child's energy system and, therefore, overall health and development. The purpose of the method is not for parents to act as clinicians and therapists. Instead, it aims to support parents and professional teams in analysing dysfunction and disease in the context of energy system health and in developing a modulation strategy that all parties understand.

Imbalances in the ESH-Prism

In Chapter 11 – *Pillar Three: Stimulation*, we discovered how the nervous and immune systems offer the most evident expression of the ESH-Triangle – creating a 'prism' for vitality. When we look at consistent imbalances that result in developmental delays or a breakdown in health, we will therefore look at them in the context of the nervous and immune systems.

Imbalances in the ESH-Prism can be mechanical, chemical, or both and manifest as:

- Neuron network imbalances (lack of pruning, lack of development, or lack of integration).
- Neuron communication imbalances (chemical and electrical).
- Gut-brain imbalances.
- Left and right brain hemisphere or area imbalances.
- Autonomic nervous system imbalances (sympathetic and parasympathetic).
- Primitive reflexes that did not integrate.
- Immune response imbalances (with a focus on inflammation).
- Metabolic and energy imbalances.

We also saw that as long as the physical structure of the prism is intact (i.e. no cell damage or obstruction), stimulation (both endo and exo) lies at the heart of the ESH-Prism equilibrium. Given that exo-stimulation (including nutrients) influences all endo-stimuli and epigenetics, and the fact that it is the only kind of stimulation we can modulate, that is where we look with the *ESH-Prism Regulation and Modulation Method* when we try to address any of the imbalances.

The ESH-Prism Regulation and Modulation Method

When there is dysfunction or illness in a child, we know that the ESH-Triangle and, therefore, ESH-Prism are out of balance. We also know that, apart from DNA and structural challenges, most imbalances start outside the body with exo-stimuli. Stimuli can be grouped as supportive stimuli, neutral stimuli and stressors. When imbalances occur, neutral stimuli may become stressors. An example of this is when a food protein starts causing sensitivities or allergies.

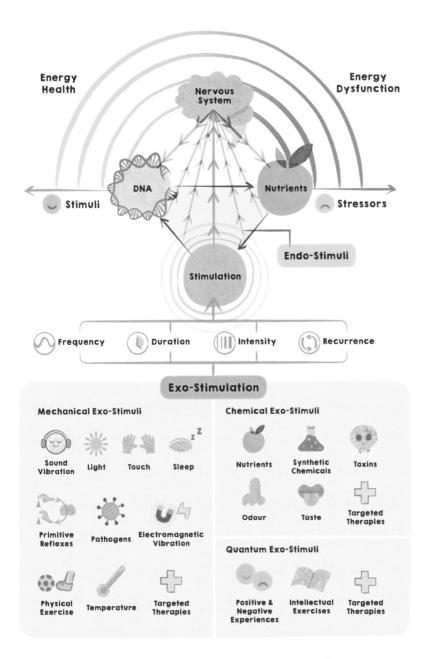

ESH-Prism Regulation and Modulation Method

The more stressors a child is exposed to without it being countered through up-regulation or down-regulation, the bigger the imbalances caused and the more unhealthy the energy system becomes. Imbalances are expressed in many developmental and illness symptoms, and even pain tolerance is affected by it. The more supportive the stimuli a child is exposed to are, the more health and development are optimised.

Regulating and Modulating Stimulation

To optimise health and development for any child, we must regulate the energy system by removing mechanical, chemical and quantum exo-stressors, encouraging the release of excessive energy from it (e.g., yawning is said to be a release valve for the autonomic nervous system) or countering their effects by adding neutral or supportive stimuli (e.g., a good night's sleep). Pain can, for example, be regulated by removing the source and or countering the pain signals by calming the autonomic nervous system. Regulation might also require controlling the frequency, intensity, duration or recurrences of certain stimuli.

Therapeutic support is, however, not only about achieving balance. Once the balance is achieved, additional supportive stimuli can be layered onto the system. This is an important step, especially when imbalances have already caused developmental delays. Stressors that should be neutral or supportive can also be reintroduced in a controlled manner, desensitising or 'inoculating' the child against the particular stimuli. This should, however, be done under clinical supervision.

Stimuli Hierarchy

As you develop your modulation strategy, it is important to know that one stimulus sometimes is reliant on another being in place for it to be effective. For example, it is no use trying to stimulate a child's cognitive development if his autonomic nervous system is out of balance. An anxious child is in fight-or-flight mode. In this stressed condition, the autonomic nervous system will take resources away from what it considers 'unessential' to survival and senses like hearing can be effective. Knowing this will help you reframe a child who appears not to listen. Or think of a malnourished child – the cognitive abilities of such a child will never be able to engage optimally if the nutritional imbalances are not corrected.

Stimuli Layering and Synergy

It is clear that imbalances, dysfunction and illness are accumulative and rarely happen in isolation. Therefore, it would also make sense to have a layered approach when it comes to modulation, therapy, and support. For the biggest impact, a collaborative approach is always encouraged by the *ESH-Prism Regulation and Modulation Method*. For optimal development and health, symptoms should never be treated in isolation – instead, their cause should be found in the ESH-Triangle. Think of a baby that suddenly struggles to fall asleep. The cause could be anything from nutrient deficiencies to room temperature.

As is the case with nutrient synergy, a particular stimulus can play a role in the effectiveness of another. Stimulating the vagus nerve in the autonomic nervous system can, for example, support an anti-inflammatory diet as it down-regulates the body. Down-regulating can also increase the production of serotonin, which can help a child sleep better. Sleep in itself is important for cell repair and growth.

Some neutral stimuli also only become stressors when others do not balance them out. Screen-time or technology on its own is not necessarily bad. It becomes an issue if too much of it results in too little movement stimuli, which are crucial for brain development.

Understanding the concept of stimuli synergy can help you evaluate treatments offered by a clinician. Think of a child that has clinical

REGULATION & MODULATION

ADHD, for example. Because medications for ADHD address the lack of dopamine, they can activate the sympathetic nervous system – making an anxious child even more anxious. Knowing this might help to incorporate therapeutic support for the increased anxiety. Another example is when too much stress plays a role in how nutrients are absorbed, which is why stressing too much about stimuli like nutrition can be counterproductive.

Priming for Stressors

In certain situations, an appropriate, controlled amount of stressors can help prime the energy system for future stressors. Here the stimuli controls play an important role. A child playing outside in the dirt is exposed to various bacteria and other pathogens. Being exposed primes the child's immune system to be 'trained' when real danger comes. The intensity of the stimuli is, however, important. One would, for example, not suggest that a child plays in sewerage to prime the immune system.

We can also prime the energy system for future stressors by stocking up on counter stimuli and illuminating as many unnecessary additional stressors as possible. Think of a child who needs surgery. Ensuring proper nutritional support and gut flora balance before and after surgery, regulating inflammation through vagus nerve stimulation, sleeping enough, and maybe rescheduling a vaccination can all counter the negative impact of surgery and promote faster healing.

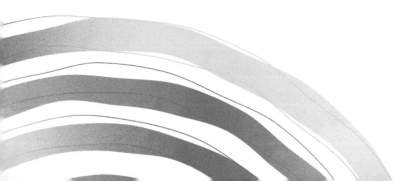

Therapy and Simulation Controls

In Chapter 3 – *The Quantum-Mechanical-Chemical Perspective,* we learned that the constructive and destructive effects of stimulation are determined by:
• Frequency (wave)
• Duration
• Intensity
• Recurrence (how often)

Therefore, a stimuli modulation strategy must consider both the objective and the controls of stimuli – specifically in the context of specialised therapeutic stimulation. Think of sound therapy. The sound frequency (Hz), how long the treatment lasts, volume and how often the treatment is given all impact the outcome – positive or negative. Red light therapy can rectify many energy system imbalances, but if any stimulation controls are wrong, it will be ineffective or even damaging. It is for this reason that modulation should be a collaboration between parents and specialists. Occupational therapy can modulate many imbalances, but one solo session a week will not do the trick – parents need to be guided in how therapy can be continued at home.

The following therapies can be applied, under specialised supervision, as part of the *ESH-Prism Regulation and Modulation Method:*
• Nutritional therapy
• Occupational therapy
• Electrotherapy
• Near-infrared light therapy
• Sound therapy
• Chiropractic therapy
• Reflexology
• Singing
• Horse riding
• Swimming

THIS LITTLE
LIGHT OF MINE

I want to end this book by reframing failures – of which I have too many to count. If we let it, a failure, like energy system imbalances, can be devastating. Failure at work or in business, an inability to stick to that diet, failure to give our children the support they need, the seeming failure of support and interventions we do provide, failure to provide a balanced meal every day, failure in relationships, failure to see warning signs and failure to know what we did not know – we all go through it, and it can all take its toll.

But I have and continue to learn that failure can also be empowering in that it 'upregulates' positive interference. It can help you to re-evaluate what to spend your precious energy on and what to avoid. It can inspire you to streamline your efforts and cancel out 'noise'. It can be a necessary stepping stone to the answers you seek and teach you to have compassion with yourself and others. It can guard you against self-centredness. It can make you brave and, to some extent, fearless!

Why is viewing failure in a balanced manner important? Raising children is rewarding, but challenging and there will be many failures. *The Firefly Theory* is not a fail-proof destination. Instead, my hope is for you to use it to facilitate and scaffold your journey in optimising your child's happiness, health and development and perhaps even your own. May this book be one of the guiding lights that helps you find your way.

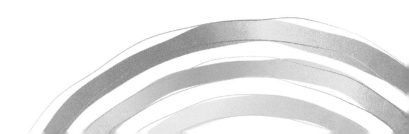

WHAT DO THE EXPERTS SAY?

"Alda Smith engages the reader through sharing her journey with her son, which sparked an investigation in important scientific pillars that will serve to inform both parents and professionals alike. A wonderful resource for families of today!" – **Maude Le Roux, Occupational Therapist, OTR/L, SIPT, Expert DIR/Floortime Training Leader, Pennsylvania, USA**

"A must for every parent with a neurodiverse child, those with neurotypical children, as well as educators, medical personnel, and support teams who need to comprehend the complexity and psychosocial dynamics that parents with these amazing children have to champion." – **Prof Pieter Fourie, M.B.Ch.B., Ph.D. (Medical Physiology), M.Med. (Paediatrics), BSc. Eng. (Electrical)**

"*The Firefly Theory* renders comprehensible, the energy system that DNA produces in concert with nutrients and our fragile environment. Smith's book will be wonderful for students of human biology, parents of neuro-diverse children and for all parents whose sense of purpose and well-being is to raise happy and healthy children." – **Susan Levine, Associate Professor of Medical Humanities, University of Cape Town**

"With her inquiring mind and fresh perspective, Alda sheds promising light on the complex interplay between health and wellness, inviting us to explore and integrate this important and fascinating field." – **Dr Mark van der Wal, Anaesthesiologist, MBBCh., father and grandfather**

"*The* parents manual to proactively raising a neurodiverse child, one pillar at a time. A must read!" – **Roberta von Meding, Mums & Tots Ireland Magazine editor & devoted mother**

"IGNITE! *The Firefly Theory* guides one through the complexity of different systems in development. It reminds us that we need to consider all of the body's systems, target intervention at the point of origin, and meet children at their unique developmental level. Most importantly, Alda highlights the need for collaboration when optimising a child's potential." – **Celette Crafford, Occupational Therapist, Sensory Integration Therapist, Advance DIR/Floortime Provider**

"*The Firefly Theory* makes so much sense from the medical point of view – the three-way balance between genetics, nutrients and stimulation is exactly what we all need."
– **Prof Steve Reid, Chair: Primary Health Care, University of Cape Town**

ACKNOWLEDGEMENTS

To my husband Johann: Thank you for our three children and a life made more beautiful by the weathering of adversity and the celebration of favour with you by my side. I wouldn't have wanted it any other way.

To my firstborn, Jesse: Thank you for making me a mother – I couldn't have asked for a kinder initiation. May you yield your gloriously sharp mind, your quick wit and open heart to a purpose bigger than yourself.

To my only daughter, Niamh: You are my drop of sweetness when life gets too bitter. Thank you for being an incredible sister, friend and teacher to Néo. What a rainbow of grace you are in his life!

To the family and 'village' on whose shoulders we rest: You know who you are. Thank you from the bottom of my heart.

To the courageous and vibrant people of South Africa: You gave me strong, purposeful roots - thank you.

To the people of Ireland: Thank you for your rich soil of opportunity.

"He drew a circle that shut me out-

Heretic, rebel, a thing to flout.

But love and I had the wit to win:

We drew a circle and took him In!"

– Edwin Markham

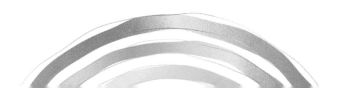

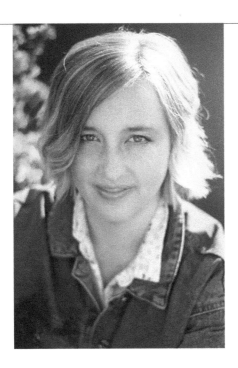

ABOUT THE AUTHOR

Alda Smith is an ordinary mum of three beautiful, diverse children, with an extraordinary narrative in medicine. As a well-published, award-winning parenting author and social advocate, Alda uses her experiences, discovery potential, and unique way of thinking to intuitively explore and understand health sciences – bridging the gap between therapists or clinicians and their patients. She has provided emotional support to over 100 women in labour and birth and has more than 500 hours of clinical observation experience – including a 20-hour-long paediatric kidney harvesting and transplant at the Netcare Christiaan Barnard Memorial Hospital in Cape Town, South Africa. She completed training in the Fundamentals of Neuroscience, has a Professional Certification in Narrative Medicine, and has completed basic overview training in photomedicine.

REFERENCES

Anderson, D., Baumgartner, A., Brunborg, G., Fthenou, E., Gdula, M., Godschalk, R., Hepworth, S., Keramarou, M., Kleinjans, J., Laubenthal, J., Poterlowicz, K., Schmid, T. Schooten, F. and Zlobinskaya, O., 2012. Cigarette smoke-induced transgenerational alterations in genome stability in cord blood of human F1 offspring. The FASEB Journal, 26(10).

Barker, R., Cicchetti, F. and Robinson, E., 2018. Neuroanatomy and neuroscience at a glance. Hoboken, NJ: John Wiley & Sons Ltd.

Bouic, P. 2020. Jonno and Prof. Patrick Bouic Talk Immunology and Nutrition in the time of the Corona. Interview with Jonno Proudfoot. Available at https://www.youtube.com/watch?v=9N6iq1qSlr0

Butterworth, C. and Tamura, T., 1989. Folic acid safety and toxicity: a brief review. The American Journal of Clinical Nutrition, 50(2), pp.353-358.

Charon, R., Gasputa, S., Hermann, N., Irvine, C., Marcus, E., Rivera Colsn, E., Spencer, D. and Spiegel, M., 2017. The principles and practice of narrative medicine. New York: Oxford University Press.

Costa, M. and Johannes, F., 2020. Epigenetics: Switching Genes On and Off. Front. Chem, 8 (554136).

Davies, S. C., 2018. Annual Report of the Chief Medical Officer, 2018 Health 2040 – Better Health Within Reach. UK: Department of Health and Social Care.

Gonzalez, G., 2012. Holographic healing. United States: Quantum Neurology Publishing.

Gutstein, S. and Gutstein, H., 2009. The RDI Book: Forging New Pathways for Autism, Asperger's and PDD with the Relationship Development Intervention Program. Houston, Tex.: Connections Center Pub.

Hutton, M., 2006. Understanding the nervous system. Scientific Pub Ltd.

Jianqin, S., Leiming, X., Lu, X., Yelland, G., Ni, J. and Clarke, A., 2015. Effects of milk containing only A2 beta casein versus milk containing both A1 and A2 beta casein proteins on gastrointestinal physiology, symptoms of discomfort, and cognitive behavior of people with self-reported intolerance to traditional cows' milk. Nutrition Journal, 15(1).

Know, L., 2018. Mitochondria and the future of medicine: the key to understanding disease, chronic illness, aging, and life itself. White River Junction, Vermont: Chelsea Green Publishing.

Levi-Montalcini, R., 2006. Neurological Disorders: Public Health Challenges. Geneva (WHO).

Lipton, B.H., 2015. The biology of belief: unleashing the power of consciousness, matter & miracles. Carlsbad, California: Hay House, Inc.

Liu, T., 2018. The scientific hypothesis of an "energy system" in the human body. Journal of Traditional Chinese Medical Sciences, 5(1), pp.29-34.

Mason, S.A., Welch, V.G. and Neratko, J. 2018. Synthetic Polymer Contamination in Bottled Water, Front. Chem, 6(407).

Melillo, R., 2015. Disconnected Kids. New York: Penguin Publishing Group.

Metropulos, M. 2017. The benefits and risks of A2 milk. Medical News Today, July 25.

Nedley, N., 2020. Crossing the Blood Brain Barrier: What Nutrients Does My Brain Need? Interview with Nathan Nedley - Nedley Health Solutions. Available at: https://www.youtube.com/watch?v=8hlC_6GBrnw.

Nemechek, P.M. and Nemechek, J.R. 2017. The Nemechek Protocol for autism and developmental disorders: a how-to guide to restoring neurological function. Buckeye, Arizona: Autonomic Recovery, Llc.

Niessen, K., Xu, M., George, D., Chen, M., Ferré-D'Amaré, A., Snell, E., Cody, V., Pace, J., Schmidt, M. and Markelz, A., 2019. Protein and RNA dynamical fingerprinting. Nature Communications, 10(1026).

Peate, I. and Gormley-Fleming, E., 2015. Fundamentals of Children's Anatomy and Physiology. West Sussex: John Wiley & Sons, Ltd.

Shanker, S. and Barker, T. 2016. Self-Reg: How to Help Your Child (and You) Break the Stress Cycle and Successfully Engage with Life. London: Yellow Kite.

Slote, C., Luu, A. and George, N.M., 2019. Ways You Can Protect Your Genes From Mutations With a Healthy Lifestyle. Front. Chem, 7(46).

Wallace, T.C., 2017. Improving nutrient absorption from food. America's Favourite Food Scientist, April 19.

Whitten, A., 2018. The Ultimate Guide to Red Light Therapy. Archangel Ink.

Winters, N. and Kelley, J.H, 2017. The metabolic approach to cancer: integrating deep nutrition, the ketogenic diet, and nontoxic bio-individualized therapies. White River Junction, Vermont: Chelsea Green Publishing.

2021. World Health Organisation. February 2021. https://www.who.int

2021. Center for Food Safety. February 2021. https://www.centerforfoodsafety.org/

Lightning Source UK Ltd.
Milton Keynes UK
UKHW020753281021
392935UK00001B/24